Concepts of Sexual Health Sex & You!

Leader's Guide
with Journal Questions

Integrating
Love & Life at the Movies: Growing in Love with the Film Classics
Roman Holiday Love and Responsibility
Educational Guidance Institute, Front Royal, VA

Concepts of Truth, Inc.
PO Box 1438
Wynne, Arkansas
info@conceptsoftruth.org
870.238.4329

ISBN: 978-0-9849652-7-4

Concepts of Sexual Health Sex & You!

TABLE OF CONTENTS

Concepts of Sexual Health Sex & You!
Overview & Rationale

The purpose of the curriculum (whether teaching live or using digital format) is to teach that the human person exists as a multidimensional being and that one's sexuality is integrated into all the dimensions. As human beings, we have the capacity to reason, make choices, seek what is true, and to ask questions of ultimate significance. The lessons in the curriculum stress that one's sexual health depends on the choice to save sex for marriage or one monogamous bond and by making healthy choices in relationships, love, and responsibility. These choices affect the whole person's present and future well-being and the heritage passed on to future generations.

According to the Arkansas State Health profile (*at the time of print- insert applicable state/country's STD stats*): http://www.cdc.gov/nchhstp/stateprofiles/pdf/arkansas_profile.pdf, Arkansas ranks eighth for Chlamydia and sixth for Gonorrheal infections in the United States.[1] Since sex involves one's sexuality, is more than an isolated act, is more than a bodily function, is not just a commodity to buy or sell, and since contraceptives do not always provide protection against STDs, sexual health education must appeal to the dispositions of the mind, heart, will, and conscience of the learner. Young people can be reached through their hearts and challenged to become persons of character, capable of contributing not only to their own well-being but also to their communities and society.

The Whole Person Learning Theory by Onalee McGraw, Ph.D., founder of the Educational Guidance Institute, Inc. and author of *Teaching the Whole Person about Love, Sex, and Marriage Educating for Character in the Common World of our Homes, Schools, and Communities*, explains the philosophical and psychological concepts of the whole person approach to learning: the philosophy that one's sexuality is an integral part of the whole person. *"As whole persons, men and women possess a sexuality that is integrated in body, mind, heart, will, and conscience. The sexual domain is permeated by the intellectual, moral, emotional, physical, and social domains. The psychological guiding principle is that cognitive powers of memory, thought, judgment, imagination, and learning related to sexuality permeate the body, mind, heart, will, and conscience; thinking, feeling, and acting in the sexual domain reflect the whole person."*[2] The premise of the whole person learning theory is foundational for *Concepts of Sexual Health Sex and You!*

The resources included in *Concepts of Sexual Health Sex and You!* are based on medical facts, statistics from the Center for Disease Control & Prevention/cdc.gov, and are developmentally appropriate for 9-12th grades.[3]

In six 90-minute lessons (or twelve 45 min. lessons) using video, powerpoint, lecture and discussion (whether using *Concepts of Sexual Health Sex & You!* digital curriculum available online or as a classroom teacher) *Concepts of Sexual Health Sex and You!* presents students with the concepts of the whole person approach and a definition for sexual health that integrates the five dimensions of the whole person; human dignity and development; classic film lesson plans from *Love & Life at the Movies: Growing in Love with the Film Classics Roman Holiday Love & Responsibility* curriculum [4] to promote virtue and character in love and marriage; medically based facts about STDs, contraception, and prevention of disease; and practical help from *The High Cost of Free Love*, Pam Stenzel[5] to guide young people in the present and future when seeking answers to life's most difficult questions. Acquiring this knowledge and life skills will give students the opportunity to pass on sexual health and a heritage for life to future generations.

For the Teacher Lesson I
Concepts of Sexual Health Sex & You!

The lesson begins with building rapport with students. Josh McDowell says, *"Rules without relationships = rebellion."*[6] Building relationships with students will produce more positive outcomes with the curriculum. Students don't care how much you know until they know how much you care. Show your passion for the subject matter! Mutual respect opens the door to hearts and lives. The lesson gives the student a glance at their preferred future and also the kind of heritage they may want to pass down to future generations. Applying the five interactive dimensions of the whole person - physical, social, emotional, intellectual, and moral, students will gain knowledge and understanding of their sexual health lived out in true freedom with purity, integrity, and unconditional love. The lesson also helps students to consider long term academic, vocational and social goals, which are a critical factor in helping teens avoid negative pressures toward sexual activity outside of marriage or one monogamous bond. *Concepts of Sexual Health Sex & You!* lessons help students consider their life's purpose, goals and to consider their complex whole being by making healthy choices in relationships, love, and responsibility.

Lesson I Objectives:
1) Teachers and students will develop a rapport by getting acquainted allowing each one to tell a few interests of sports, hobbies, etc. with at least 90% participation from class.
2) Participants will be able to define sexual health and describe the purpose of sex in relation to the five interactive dimensions of the whole person, i.e., physical, emotional, intellectual, social and moral with 75% participation.
3) By comparing risky sexual behaviors outside of one monogamous bond, students will be able to list benefits of integrity, purity and unconditional love within the five interactive dimensions of the whole person. During lecture, ppt presentation, discussion and writing in journals, students will give an acceptable range of answers that are allowable as correct. (If using *Concepts of Sexual Health Sex & You!* digital online curriculum lessons, teachers can stop and discuss.)
4) Students will be given the opportunity to evaluate their own sexual health in relation to the whole person concept with at least 50% of class participation.

Lesson Plan

Permission is given by the authors to insert applicable substitutes for video clip/s, handouts, or slides based on current stats/population/culture maintaining the meaning and values of the original content.

Activities: Sonic Coupon Activity, 2 Paper Hearts; Duct Tape/Bonding

Distribution of Journals (If teacher is using the *Concepts of Sexual Health Sex & You!* digital online curriculum, the journal questions are included and may be recorded on student's notebook paper. The journal questions are in the teacher's manual and can be read for students to write their answers on notebook paper. Hard copy student journals are an available option and sold separately.)

Handouts: Planning the Future Checklist (Appendix Lesson 1), Handout: Secondary Virginity (Appendix Lesson 1)

Lecture & Discussion

Video: Attention Getter clip

PowerPoints (Ppt): (1) Choices, Choices (2) Integrity, Identity & Intimacy Capability (3) WHO Sexual Health Definition (4) COT's Sexual Health Definition (5) Words of Sexual Health Definition (6) The Five Aspects of the Whole Person (7) Sex & You (8) Whole Purpose of Sex (9) Science of Sex (10) Duct Tape Activity (11) Planning The Future (12) Planning Your Children's Future (13) Uniquely Different

Lesson I Classroom
Concepts of Sexual Health Sex & You!

Get Acquainted
Hello, my name is.... from (local organization.) I'm excited to be here and I look forward to getting to know you better. There is only one rule. . .I will respect you and I expect you to respect me.

No matter what you say in here, I won't treat you any differently. Now, here's a little bit about me and what I do. And, I want to learn who you are and something you are involved in or what you like to do. *(Tell a little about yourself and get to know the students/clients briefly. Have them say their names and what grade they are in, if they play sports, band, etc. Building a relationship with them is very important!)*

Introduction
This class will meet once a week for six weeks (note 12 weeks if class is 45 min.) It will help you to live out your sexuality in true freedom with integrity, purity and unconditional love. The lessons are a plan for individuals and families to live sexually healthy and whole without regret and to pass on a wonderful heritage to future generations.

This class will help you consider the five interactive dimensions or aspects of a whole person while making healthy choices in relationships, love, and responsibility. It will give you tools that will last for a lifetime, a way to discover and keep, not only your true love, but a purpose for your life. This class is called *Concepts of Sexual Health Sex & You!* You'll find this curriculum is not an abstinence program. But it is about your sexuality being interconnected to your whole person. Finding sexual health through purity and choosing to save sex for one monogamous bond is **not merely about saying "no" to sexual activity but about saying "yes" to love and responsibility**. Sexual Health is about **YOU** - your <u>whole</u> self.

We will have lots of videos and powerpoints and even teach you how to twerk! (**Short video clip for attention getter**). But first, let's start with a checklist that will help you plan for your future and for your children's future. There is no right or wrong answer and this will not be graded.

Handout: Planning The Future Checklist *(Ask for a few students to share their answers – several will probably have checked all items. Talk about how we all desire good, whole, pure things for our future and how we all want to leave behind a good example/heritage for our children.)*

Sonic Coupon Activity:
Basically, we all want good things. How many of you would like a good thing like a free sonic coupon? Remember when you were in elementary school wanting to be chosen for a certain team game or sport? *(As hands are raised, leader will take some time in choosing a recipient. Walk around, scratch your head, maybe have a couple to stand up and compare shirts, shoes etc. Tell them you like or dislike something about them and finally choose one or more to receive a coupon and tell the others you are sorry they were not included in your choice.)*

Lesson 1 Classroom Continued

We make choices every day and **choices have consequences**! Some consequences are good and some are bad. As a leader, I just made a choice as to who would receive these free coupons and the consequence happened to be a good one. . . someone won!

We all want to be chosen and as human persons we all have the dignity and deserve the right to be chosen! We all have a need to be liked, included, and desired. We value good things. In our inner core is the natural human desire to give and receive unconditional love. We long for love, relationships and of course. . .free things. . .like these sonic coupons! (*Give away one or more coupons.*)

The things we desire and can choose in life are both tangible (*can see*) and intangible (*can't see*). They include things like someone to love us unconditionally, a fairy tale romance, good jobs, nice homes, adventure, happiness, peace, and contentment.

Unfortunately, our choices do not always produce the desired outcome or positive consequences. Sometimes in life we think we're headed in the right direction, only to find the choice we took led us to pain and heartbreak. Have you looked at any magazines or celebrity news shows lately?

They are full of stories of people (give examples of famous people) who may be married for years and now divorcing. Or people that don't get married at all - like friends with benefits or the hook up. They just cruise from one person to another – one bed to another. These are people who seem to make poor choices and end up getting hurt.

The next powerpoint shows a person trying to choose. . .if only we could look ahead and see inside the treasure chest!

Ppt 1, Lesson 1

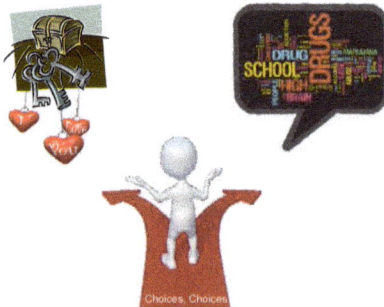

Lesson 1 Classroom Continued

Is the romance of Cinderella and her Prince just a fairy tale, or is it possible to find the one true love of your life. . .and keep them? Fortunately, there is! There is a way to find true love, true freedom, sexual purity, and a way to make healthy choices in relationships, love, and responsibility.

One can have sexual health as a whole person and know a relationship based on unconditional, committed married love. In her book, *Teaching the Whole Person about Love, Sex and Marriage, Educating for Character in the Common World of our Homes, Schools, and Communities,* author Onalee McGraw, Ph.D lists three areas of **integrity**, **identity**, and **intimacy**[7] that can be achieved by "*all persons through their natural human capacities of reason, desire for the good, voluntary will and moral sense.*" [8]

She says this can "**be true for all** *persons regardless of their own particular family background, the community where they live, or the cultural era in which they come of age.*"[9]

Ppt 2, Lesson 1

(A human person has)

The capacity to develop and maintain a core Integrity.

The capacity to form a whole person Identity.

The capacity to create true Intimacy.

(**Source:** Onalee McGraw, *Teaching the Whole Person About Love, Sex & Marriage* (2004), 52.)

You'll find this ppt. and other information in your Student Journal. (If teacher is using the *Concepts of Sexual Health Sex & You!* digital online curriculum, the journal questions are included and may be recorded on student's notebook paper. The journal questions are in the teacher's manual and can be read for students to write their answers on notebook paper. Hard copy student journals are an available option and sold separately.)

Pass out Journals (If using hard copy option) These Journals are your private property. They are a gift from *(whoever purchased them).* They cost about $5.00 each and will not be replaced during this six-week period. Please keep up with them, protect them, bring them to class, and record your answers and thoughts in them. Someday you will want to look back and see how you answered some of life's most important questions and also your answers can be a current resource to you!

Also, the class that has the most participation in bringing back the journals will have a great reward. . .coupons. . .coupons!

Lesson 1 Classroom Continued

What is Sexual Health?

Ppt 3, Lesson 1

What is Sexual Health?
(World Health Organization definition)
Sexual Health is.........
a state of physical, emotional, mental and social well-being. In relation to sexuality; it is not merely the absence of disease, dysfunction, or infirmity. Sexual health requires a positive and respectful approach to sexuality and sexual relationships, as well as the possibility of having pleasurable and safe sexual experiences, free of coercion, discrimination, and violence.

The "**WHO (World Health Organization) working definition 2002** (says): *Sexual health is a state of physical, emotional, mental and social well-being. In relation to sexuality; it is not merely the absence of disease, dysfunction, or infirmity. Sexual health requires a positive and respectful approach to sexuality and sexual relationships, as well as the possibility of having pleasurable and safe sexual experiences, free of coercion, discrimination, and violence.*"

According to research on sexually transmitted diseases and the fact that one's sexuality is interconnected and integrated throughout the whole person, we cannot have a safe sexual experience except in the bonds of one monogamous partner expressing unconditional love.

Our sexual health depends upon living out our sexuality in true freedom and wholeness, which involves the five dimensions or aspects of the whole person. Let's learn a definition for sexual health based on the whole person concept.

Ppt 4, Lesson 1

(Concepts of Truth's Definition)
Sexual Health is.........
living out one's sexuality in true freedom with integrity, purity and unconditional love.

It is making healthy choices in relationships, love and responsibility that will affect the whole person present and future and the heritage passed on to future generations.

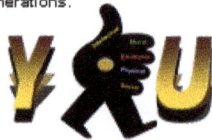

Concepts of Truth's definition for Sexual Health based on the whole person concept:
Sexual health is living out one's sexuality in true freedom with integrity, purity and unconditional love. It is making healthy choices in relationships, love, and responsibility that will affect the whole person present and future and the heritage passed on to future generations.

Lesson 1 Classroom Continued

Anyone who can learn Concepts of Truth's Sexual Health definition word for word by the end of the six weeks will be eligible to be in a drawing for free movie tickets! Now, let's break down the definition and explore the meaning of each word in the following powerpoint:

Ppt 5, Lesson 1
(Have students read & discuss)

Sexual:	Relating to, or associated with sex or the sexes, male & female
Health:	The condition of being sound in body, mind, or spirit; *especially* : freedom from physical disease or pain
True:	Honest, consistent, ideal
Freedom:	The quality or state of being free: as the absence of necessity, coercion, or constraint in choice or action. Freedom involves a choice.
Integrity:	The quality or state of being complete or undivided; unbroken ; wholeness; entirety; being unimpaired; perfect condition; soundness; being of sound moral principle; uprightness, honesty, and sincerity, firm adherence to a code especially moral, ethic, or artistic.
Purity:	Freedom from adulterating matter; cleanness or clearness freedom from evil or improper motives; innocence; chastity
Unconditional Love:	Not conditional or limited; absolute, unqualified, *unconditional* surrender, synonyms: perfect, pure, total unadulterated
	Definitions from www.merriam-webster.com/dictionary

To have true freedom, integrity and purity in sexual health means to consistently live our lives with the highest moral sexual standards and unconditional love consistently guarding your mind, will and emotions from sexual impurity. To live sexually healthy **is to be the same in the dark as you are in the light**. To have sexual health means we set limits on how much of our bodies we share with others. Sexual health is possible for anyone, regardless of past choices or painful experiences.

Question: What are your dreams and goals for your sexual health?

Sex & You!

Sex is not an isolated act. It is not about *doing* but it is about *being* male or female. Sex is you - the whole person! Our sexuality is interconnected and integrated throughout the whole person and affects us intellectually, morally, emotionally, physically and socially. Sex is more than a bodily function and not just a commodity to buy or sell.

Contraceptives do not always provide protection against STDs so sexual health education must appeal to dispositions of the mind, heart, will, and conscience of the learner. In her book, *Teaching the Whole Person About Love, Sex & Marriage*, author Onalee McGraw, PhD describes **The Five Aspects of the Whole Person**.

Lesson 1 Classroom Continued

She says, *"Life is experienced on many levels. In our attitudes, relationships and behavior we all experience life as whole persons. In human life, our reason, moral sense and emotions, our bodies and our social relationships are all in play simultaneously. Furthermore, each of these domains is affected by the others. The human person must always be considered as a whole person - never in parts."*

(You can give an example using a baby crib mobile or anything that could represent a system all working together. When one part moves, it affects the other parts because it is part of the whole operating system.)

Ppt 6, Lesson 1
(read slide)

The Whole Person

Intellectual
Human persons possess an intellect enabling them to think and grasp abstract ideas, and a will enabling them to make rational choices.

↓

Moral
Our intellects enable us to recognize the distinction between good and evil, right and wrong. Our will is then confronted with the task of living accordingly.

↓   ↓

Emotions and Feelings	**Physical**
Emotions and feelings permeate our whole person. Mature persons have the ability to control their emotions, subjecting them to intellectual and moral standards.	The body is the living organism that houses each of us. Ideally, our physical actions will be controlled by properly ordered emotional responses, but since the body sometimes matures more quickly than the intellect and the emotions, this is not always easy.

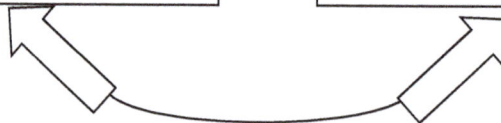

Social

Each person is part of a community. As we grow we learn to interact with others, develop friendships and work to benefit others as well as ourselves.[11]

Lesson 1 Classroom Continued

Let's remember the whole person on our five fingers. The five aspects are intellectual, moral, emotional, physical and social. Give your neighbor a "high five".

Ppt 7, Lesson 1

Sex and YOU!

The human person is uniquely intricate and whole. Our body, mind, heart, will, emotions and our social and moral sense function integratively to make us who we are.

Our sexuality is an integral part of our entire being and our unique and personal inner core. In this inner core is the natural human desire to give and receive unconditional love.

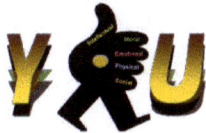

The human person is uniquely intricate and whole. Our body, mind, heart, will, emotions and our social and moral sense function together and are integrated to make us who we are.

Our sexuality is an integral part of our entire being and our unique and personal inner core. In this inner core is the natural human desire to give and receive unconditional love. So, now we have the title of this program, *Concepts of Sexual Health Sex & You!*

If Sex is Not an Act, What is the Purpose?
J. Budziszewski, professor of Government & Philosophy, University of Texas, Austin paints the following scenario in his article, *"What We Lose When We Forget What Sex Is For"*:

"**Midnight**. Shelly is getting herself drunk so that she can bring herself to go home with the strange man seated next to her at the bar. **One o'clock**. Steven is busy downloading pornographic images of children from internet bulletin boards. **Two o'clock**. Marjorie, who used to spend every Friday night in bed with a different man, has been binging and purging since eleven. **Three o'clock**. Pablo stares through the darkness at the ceiling wondering how to convince his girlfriend to have an abortion. **Four o'clock**. After partying all night, Jesse takes another man home, not mentioning that he tests positive for an incurable STD. **Five o'clock**. Lisa is in the bathroom, cutting herself delicately with a razor. This isn't what my generation expected when it invented the sexual revolution. The game isn't fun anymore. Even some of the diehard proponents of that enslaving liberation have begun to show signs of fatigue and confusion."[12]

Lesson 1 Classroom Continued

Ppt 8, Lesson 1

Y♥U

WHOLE
Purpose of
SEX

Procreation
Bonding/Unitive Intimacy
Completion
Marital & Family Life

Source: J. Budziszewski "What We Loose When We Forget What Sex Is For"

The WHOLE Purpose of Sex
Sex is for procreation, bonding/unitive intimacy, completion, marital & family life. . .and yes, it is pleasurable!
Sex between a male and female (*complementary opposites*) brings a man and woman together in unitive intimacy. J. Budziszewski says, *"...the longing for unitive intimacy is at the center of our design."* [13]

In the research study report, *"Hardwired to Connect: The New Scientific Case for Authoritative Communities."* 2003 issued by the Commission on Children at Risk, the authors state there are two kinds of connectedness: *close connections to other people, and deep connections to moral and spiritual meaning.* Plank #10 states *"The human brain appears to be organized to ask ultimate questions, and seek ultimate answers.*[14]

We all long for the purpose of sex - transcendent, unconditional love, connecting to the opposite sex and producing children as a symbol for this union of completeness.

Pleasure is a byproduct of sex, but not the ultimate goal. Pleasure comes naturally as a byproduct of pursuing something else. For instance, the purpose of eating is for nutrition but eating is pleasurable. If we ate simply for pleasure it would be unhealthy. If we use sex simply for pleasure someone gets used. It becomes selfish and disordered.

Sex is for procreation (*producing children*), **unity, completeness and family life**. And outside of celibacy (abstaining from sexual intercourse, especially by reason of religious vows, unmarried) there is something missing in the man, which must be provided by the woman and vice versa. **Men and women complement each other**. The book *Men are Like Waffles, Women are Like Spaghetti* [15]is a good resource to explain the complementary relationship.

Again, referring to the article *"What We Lose When We Forget What Sex Is For"* there is a "**natural law of sex**".[16] Physically, in order to procreate a man and woman need each other. But also, we long for the unitive intimacy in a relationship based on unconditional love.

Lesson 1 Classroom Continued

Marriage and family life are part of natural law. There is never a time in human history when they did not exist. According to the Universal Declaration of Human Rights, the family is the natural and fundamental group unit of society and is entitled to protection by society and the State.[17] We are not designed for "hooking up", but we are designed for our bodies and our hearts to work together.

The ideology of hooking up says that sex is merely release or recreation. Author J. Budziszewski goes on to say, *"Mutual and total self-giving strong feelings of attachment, intense pleasure, and the procreation of new life are linked by human nature in a single complex of purpose. If it is true that they are linked by human nature, then if we try to split them apart, we split ourselves."*[18]

In your journal on Pg. 6, you will find the following statement by J. Budziszewski. Let's say it together. (*It almost sounds like the old Peter Piper Picked a Peck of Pickled Peppers rhyme!*) **"The gift of self makes each self to the other self what no other self can be".**[19] (*Have students try saying it faster just for fun and to help them remember the phrase.*)

To "forsake all others" is not just a sentimental feature of traditional Western marriage vows; it arises from the very nature of the gift. You cannot partly give yourself, because yourself is indivisible as a whole person; **the only way to give yourself is to give yourself entirely.**

Because the gift is total, it has to exclude all others, and if it doesn't do that, then it hasn't taken place.[20] Sex involves the whole person. Our sexuality is a gift to be given with unconditional love. It is a whole act with a **WHOLE PURPOSE.**

(Note: 45-minute class time end here.)

Lesson 1 Classroom Continued (Note: 45-minute class time begin here)

Activity: Paper Hearts (*Prior to class, cut out 3 hearts-2 of one color, and one of another color.   Pre-glue one of each color together before the presentation. At the beginning of the presentation hold up the glued hearts showing one side with the different color from the single heart color, and the single heart of the other color and explain the following scenario as an object lesson:*)
(Note: In order to be more relevant for high school students, it is suggested to add that Dan and Jan were in high school and that their relationship lasted only the average of 3 weeks after having sex.) (This scenario is used by permission and found in the book *The Invisible Bond* by Barbara Wilson.)[21]

"Dan and Jan thought they were in love. Even though they didn't want to have sex, they hadn't made any previous decisions about sexual intimacy and didn't set mutually agreed-upon boundaries. Their passion snuck up on them, they got carried away, and....it happened. (*staple the single heart to the same color side of the glued heart representing the bonding that occurs not letting the audience see the glued side so they think you've just stapled them together.*)

When we have a sexual relationship with someone, the bonding is not just physical. It affects the whole person. What we are really looking for when having sex outside of marriage is true intimacy - interpersonal communication at the deepest level.

We look to sex to provide the closeness and love that we're longing for. The bonding happens whether one is married or not. Sex makes us feel close even when we hardly know each other. Yet couples who initiate sex early on in a relationship have difficulty moving to that deepest level and experiencing true intimacy with each other."

Finally, Dan and Jan break up. (*Rip the two hearts that were glued to signify Dan and Jan's break up.*) And, to their surprise, a piece of their heart is left behind. Each leaving pieces still attached to the other. Neither heart came away whole.

The Science of Sex
A "science of sex" occurs when bonding hormones oxytocin and vasopressin are released during the act of intercourse. [22] This bonding is not outwardly seen but inwardly expressed.

Ppt 9, Lesson 1

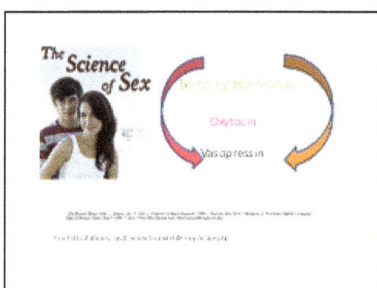

Lesson 1 Classroom Continued

During sexual activity, these powerful hormones are released in the brains of men and women that produce lasting bonds with their partner. Oxytocin is a bonding hormone released during childbirth and nursing that causes the mother to bond with her infant.

It is also released during sexual activity and acts as emotional super glue between partners. Both men and women have oxytocin and release it during sexual activity; but women are more affected by oxytocin and men by vasopressin, another bonding hormone released during sex.

Vasopressin helps a man bond to his partner and instills a protective instinct toward his partner and children.

Ppt 10, Lesson 1

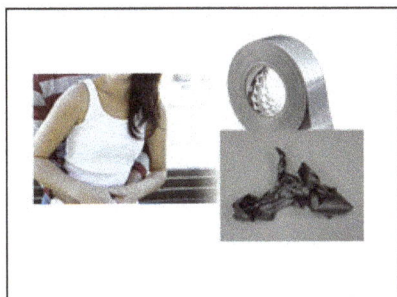

Duct Tape Activity

(Wrap duct tape around your arm and the arm of your co-facilitator.)
When a couple has sex the bonding hormones are released so the tape is tight. Sex is like adhesive. Promiscuity is like taking the tape off again and again. We want to be bonded forever with one monogamous partner to live happily ever after.

(Now take the tape off and try to stick the same tape a second time.) This represents the couple deciding to have different sexual partners. There are pieces of skin cells, hair, etc. on the tape and it won't stick as good the second time without problems. **The choice to have more than a permanent, monogamous relationship creates problems intellectually, morally, emotionally, physically, and socially.**

Research suggests the ability to bond and produce oxytocin is damaged by the stress hormones released during a breakup. Just like debris on duct tape, previous sexual experiences reduce the ability to bond correctly. Oxytocin levels can return to normal if sexual activity is stopped and time is given to address physical and emotional healing.

Lesson 1 Classroom Continued

Refrain from getting into a new relationship for a year or two and commit to save sex for marriage. Secondary Virginity is possible. How many have ever heard of that term before? If you have already had sex, that doesn't mean that you have to continue. You can stop now, allow your body and emotions to heal and save your gift for one monogamous partner. Let's look briefly at what secondary virginity means.

Handout: Secondary Virginity [23] (*Appendix, Lesson 1- give overview of the concept of secondary virginity, tell students to read through after class.*)

Imagine the duct tape was never removed. The duct tape would begin to feel like a part of the arm and the adhesion would be strong. **When a couple waits until marriage to have sex and remains faithful to each other during the marriage, oxytocin and vasopressin increase the biological bond between the husband and wife.**[24]

Remember... the definition of sexual health includes true freedom that will affect the future! Having sexual health is for a lifetime! It continues even after marriage.

Question: Explain the **WHOLE** Purpose of Sex:

Question: Are you living out your sexuality with sexual health or secondary virginity? Explain.

Planning the Future
Have you chosen to have premarital sex? This choice allows risks in all areas of your life, because you are a whole person.

Couples who cohabitate (*live together before marriage*) also increase their risks of damage to their sexual health. Let's read the risks listed in the Intellectual, Moral, Emotional, Physical, and Social dimensions:[25]

Lesson 1 Classroom Continued

Ppt 11, Lesson 1
(Note: Intellectual, Moral, Emotional, Physical and Social will come up individually on the powerpoint with examples. This powerpoint and the next one are important parts of the first lesson. Take time to discuss each part.)

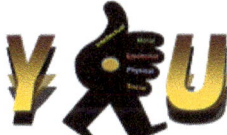

Planning Your Children's Future

If you have chosen to have premarital sex, that choice will not only affect your future but will also have an impact on your children's future. What kind of future do you want for them? Read what your children may experience in the five dimensions of the whole person.

Ppt 12, Lesson 1
(Note: Emotional, Intellectual, Moral, Physical and Social will come up individually on the powerpoint with examples. This powerpoint and the next one is an important part of this first lesson. Take time to discuss each part.)

Question: Think about your recent choices. How have your choices affected your whole person?

Ppt 13, Lesson 1

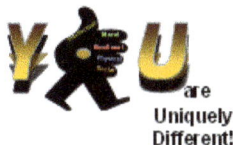

Uniquely Different!
There is no one in the world just like you! Your DNA, fingerprints, your hand clap, the pitch of your voice are all unique. Remember, men and women are uniquely different not only as male and female but as our individual self. Male and female are unique individuals with different roles that complement the other.

In the book *Men Are Like Waffles, Women Are Like Spaghetti* [26] by Bill and Pam Farrel, we find that most women can multi-task and be everywhere at the same time, like spaghetti. Most women can talk on the phone and plan their grocery list while painting their nails; whereas men usually focus on one item at a time.

Most men are innately protective and secure like a box in the waffle. Women usually talk more, share feelings more easily, and typically are more nurturing and emotional than men. Men are innately protectors and usually take more time in making decisions so the analogy of staying in one box, completing the task before moving on to another. So, men and women complement each other. Understanding these concepts will help your relationships now and in the future.

Question: Do you agree with the phrase *Men are like Waffles and Women are like Spaghetti?*
Among your friends and family, how have you seen this phrase demonstrated?

Resources
Book: Men Are Like Waffles, Women Are Like Spaghetti
Bill and Pam Farrel
Website for Parents: www.concernedparents.com

For the Teacher Lesson 2 Concepts
Development & Dignity

In this lesson, students will explore fertility, prenatal development and the dignity of all human persons. All human life has value and our fertility gives us the power to create human life. The more teens understand the development and unique dignity of a human person, the intrinsic value of life and the gift of fertility, the more they will be empowered in relationships to make healthy reproductive choices.

Students will also explore the *Universal Declaration of Human Rights* in the context of love, sexuality and relationships. They will examine the premise that our bodies and our sexuality are an integral part of our unique and personal inner core. In this inner core is the natural human desire to give and receive unconditional love. Using video and models, they will view prenatal development and analyze the human life cycle from fertilization to infancy and their ability to create human life.

Objectives:

1) Students will compare and contrast male and female reproductive organs exploring the power of fertility and be able to describe that responsibility in sexual decisions with 75% of students participating in discussion.

2) Students will view the video TED: *Alexander Tsiaras The Ink Conference* and a set of pre-natal models representing human development from 7- 30 weeks gestation. Students will be able to identify the stages of human development and describe the characteristics of each stage using the pre/post test questions with at least 75% accuracy.

3) By discussing the acrostic *S.L.E.D.*, students will be able to compare and contrast the four differences between the preborn and born human person and apply the concepts in future situations when defending the true value and dignity of the human person with 50% participation from the class.

4) Students will be able to define intrinsic and extrinsic value and apply the definition to love and responsibility in relationships sexuality with 75% participation and accuracy.

Lesson Plan

Permission is given by the authors to insert applicable substitutes for video clip/s, handouts, or slides based on current stats/population/culture maintaining the meaning and values of the original content.

Activity: $20 Bill (Giving Value & Dignity To A Human Person)

Handouts: TED: Alexander Tsiaras The Ink Conference Pre/Post Test Questions (with answer key in Appendix Lesson 2)

Touch of Life Fetal Models

Journal Pages

Lecture & Discussion

PowerPoints (Ppt): (1) Male & Female Fertility (2) Horton (3-9) S.L.E.D. (10) Universal Declaration of Human Rights (11) The Dignity of a Human Person (12) Outward & Inward Dignity (13) Inward Dignity & You (14) Applying Extrinsic Value to Relationships (15) Applying Intrinsic Value to Relationships (16) Unconditional Love (17) Whole Person

Video: TED: Alexander Tsiaras (2010 Partner) The Ink Conference[27] (10 min.) Image-maker Alexander Tsiaras shares a powerful medical visualization, showing human development from conception to birth and beyond.

Lesson 2 Classroom
Development & Dignity

Introduction:

Today, we will explore the power of fertility, prenatal development, and the dignity of all human persons. We will look at the Universal Declaration of Human Rights in the context of love, sexuality and relationships. **How does sex result in procreation? What does it mean to be a whole person? Does human life have dignity (a presence that commands respect) and value**? Let's read the following ppt:

Ppt No. 1, Lesson 2

Male & Female Fertility

Both the male and female brain stimulates the pituitary gland.

The pituitary gland stimulates the testes in the male & ovaries in the female.

The testes produce sperm and produce the hormone testosterone. The ovaries release the ova (eggs) and produce the hormones estrogen and progesterone.

Most male reproductive organs are outside the body and most female reproductive organs are inside, needing protection.

Men do not produce sperm until puberty. From puberty on, the male body will produce hundreds of thousands of sperm every day until the man dies.

Girls are born with all the eggs they will ever have. Upon puberty, girls begin to release one egg per cycle.(Approximately one per month) Women stop releasing eggs mid-life (late 40's or 50's) and undergo menopause.

While a man's hormones are normally balanced, a woman's varies during her cycle.

Fertility, the Beginning

Our fertility gives us power to create human life. Fertility is the state of or being fertile and fertile means one is capable of reproducing. The male and female are complementary to each other. Females have open reproductive systems and male have closed. The female provides the egg (ovum) with 23 chromosomes, the male fertilizes with his sperm of 23 chromosomes and the female incubates the resulting zygote with 46 chromosomes (*Human DNA genetic code*).

Procreation also requires an enduring partnership between two beings. Why would both parents be needed? To raise the child, both are needed because the male is innately the protector and the female the nurturer. A parent of each sex is necessary to make the child, to raise the child and to teach the child.

The child needs a model of his own sex, a model of the other and a model of the relationship between them. The partnership in procreation continues even after the children are grown, because then they (the parents) are needed to help them (the children) establish their own new families.[28]

Question:

Fertility - Understanding our fertility, helps us make healthier choices in relationships and reproductive choices. If you don't have a committed relationship with someone and you are having sex with them, you risk choosing them as the mother or father for your child. Write your thoughts about your fertility.

Lesson 2 Classroom Continued

Becoming A Whole Person.
In Lesson One, we looked at a human being as a whole person. In our human nature, our body, mind, will, emotions, as well as social and moral senses, function together to make us who we are.

Popular media often judge the whole person by appearance or by what one can or cannot do. **This view of the whole person reduces us as objects to be used**.

Some believe a person isn't a person until after birth. Even Dr. Seuss has an opinion! Do you know what he says about a person? In *Horton Hears a Who*, Horton says, *"And, even though you can't hear them or see them at all, a person's a person, no matter how small."*[29]

Ppt. No. 2, Lesson 2

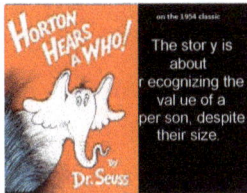

Handout: Pre/Post Questions for Video -Ted: Alexander Tsiaras

Please answer the Pre/Post Test questions before we watch the video and then afterwards we will see how well you listened by going over the answers.

The video will share a powerful medical visualization, showing human development from conception to birth and beyond. (**Show Video** – *TED: Alexander Tsiaras*[30] (10 min.)

Let's check the answers on Pre/Post Test and see how well you listened.

(Display Touch of Life Fetal Models [31]12-30 weeks gestation)
Let's take a few minutes to pass around these fetal models so you can get a more real tangible picture of prenatal development.

Question:
How and when do you define a whole person? Before or after birth; by what one can do or what one looks like? Do we wait until a month after the baby is born or can we define the fetus in the womb?

Lesson 2 Classroom Continued

J

Question: Based on the information you have seen and heard today, do you agree with Horton in Horton Hears A Who? Why or Why not?

Ppt. 3, Lesson 2

SLED

S.L.E.D.
Bio ethicist Scott Klusendorf with the group Stand to Reason(str.org[32]) says that there are only 4 major differences between the baby in the womb and the newborn or toddler. He made an acrostic of the four differences and they spell SLED.

Ppt. 4, Lesson 2

Size

Level of Development

Environment

Degree of Dependency

He says that these differences can be used to educate people in the form of questions. While looking at the next powerpoint pictures, let's read the four differences asking the questions associated with each one. And ask yourself if these differences help you to understand the dignity of the unborn. Or ask yourself if killing the unborn could ever be justified.

Ppt. 5, Lesson 2 (Picture of a BB star & super model)

Size - Are small people less human than large people? Are tall people more human than short people?

Ppt. 6, Lesson 2 (*Picture of movie star & baby girl*)

Lesson 2 Classroom Continued

Level of Development - Does intelligence gain us more rights as a human? Is a 4 yr old little girl, whose reproductive system is not fully developed, less human than a grown lady?

Ppt. 7, Lesson 2 (*picture of teenager standing inside and outside*)

Environment - Does changing environments change who we are? Does getting out of a warm house and walking out into the cold weather make us less or more of a human? Does traveling 8 in. down the birth canal make the fetus more or less human?

Ppt. 8, Lesson 2 (*Picture of doctor checking possibly someone with a pace maker & dad holding newborn*)

Degree of Dependency - Are people who are dependent on insulin pumps less of a human than people who are not? Even after a baby is born he/she is dependent on the parents while it is still young. Does that dependency make the baby less human than an adult?

So, let's review the differences that spell S.L.E.D.

Ppt. 9, Lesson 2

Size

Level of Development

Environment

Degree of Dependency

(Note: 45-minute class time end here.)

Lesson 2 Classroom Continued

Giving Value & Dignity To A Human Person (Note: 45-minute class time begin here.)

Activity $20 Bill:
I have a $20 bill in my hand. How many of you would like to have it? *(Now wad the bill up, throw it on the floor and stomp on it pressing it hard and saying it isn't any good.)* Now how many of you still want it? You probably still want it because you know regardless of what it looks like, it still has value.

According to the *Universal Declaration of Human Rights*[33] *set forth on December 10, 1948 by the General Assembly of the United Nations,* human beings (*men & women*) are so valuable that we come with "human rights" already attached.

"Human rights" mean that we owe each other respect and protection for our unique intrinsic dignity. These rights are called "inalienable rights" because they cannot be removed from us by anyone. They need to be determined to promote social progress and better standards of life in larger freedom.

Article No. 1 says, all human beings are born free and equal in dignity and rights. They are endowed with reason and conscience and should act towards one another in a spirit of brotherhood.

Article No. 2 says, everyone is entitled to all the rights and freedoms set forth in this Declaration, without distinction of any kind, such as race, color, sex, language, religion, political or other opinion, national or social origin, property, birth or other status.

Article No. 3 says, everyone has the right to life, liberty and security of person.

The declaration is composed of a Preamble and 30 Articles.
Let's watch the following short clip that explains this declaration.[34]

Ppt 10, Lesson 2

Universal Declaration of Human Rights (video clip)

Question: Article No. 3 of the Universal Declaration of Human Rights says that everyone has the right to life, liberty and security of person. Which of these are most important to you? Why?

The Dignity of the Human Person

Ppt No. 11, Lesson 2

The Dignity of a Human Person

A human person has at their inner core an intrinsic value, the natural innate (inborn) desire to give and receive unconditional love . A human person is made to fulfill his/hers highest potential by developing a sense of identity, self-worth, personal insight, meaning and purpose. As humans we have self control or the power over our mind, heart and will that is kept by the ability to tell right from wrong. This gives us the ability to surrender to self and become emotionally committed to a loving and lasting monogomous relationship in marriage and express the same unconditional love we have received.

A human person has at their inner core an intrinsic value, the natural innate *(inborn)* **desire to give and receive unconditional love.**

A human person is made to fulfill his/her highest potential by developing a sense of identity, self-worth, personal insight, meaning and purpose.

As humans, we have self-control or the power over our mind, heart and will that is kept by the ability to tell right from wrong.

This gives us the ability to surrender to self and become emotionally committed to a loving and lasting monogamous relationship in marriage and express the same unconditional love we have received.

Outward or Inward Dignity

Regardless of a human being's looks, conditions, what they can or cannot do, humans have value based on their inalienable rights and this value or right to life, liberty and security of the person cannot be removed.

Giving someone value or dignity (respect) based on what they look like, what they own or what they can do is valuing a person **outwardly or extrinsically**.

Also, if we only look at a person's behavior and success in what they can do, we miss seeing who they really are on the inside.

Lesson 2 Classroom Continued

As human beings, we are whole persons. Our body, mind, will, emotions, as well as social and moral senses function together to make us who we are.

Our bodies and our sexuality are an integral part of our unique and personal inner core. In this inner core is the natural human desire to give and receive unconditional love.

When we look at the whole person and one's ability to give and receive love in the world, we see the person's **inward or intrinsic dignity**.

Ppt No. 12, Lesson 2

> **Outward & Inward Dignity**
>
> **Outward or Extrinsic Dignity:**
> Looks, material things, behaviors & successes in what one can do
>
> **Inward or Intrinsic Dignity**
> Desire & capacity to give and receive unconditional love

Valuing a person for being human and respecting them **intrinsically**, not for what material possessions they own or what they can or cannot do will help you value and respect others in your present and/or future relationships.

Question: Do you value yourself intrinsically or extrinsically?

How a person values themselves is usually the way one values others. Remember to treat others as you would want to be treated - with mutual respect and value.

In most counseling sessions, a major presenting problem of clients is low self-worth and those who cannot accept that they are unique and valuable. If you feel the same, it is important to seek help. Talk with your parents or a trusting adult, your teachers or your counselors.

Lesson 2 Classroom Continued

We are all here to help you know that **you** have intrinsic value as a human person. In your inner core is the natural human desire to give and receive unconditional love. Looks, material things or success doesn't matter and doesn't define you as a whole person. **You are a unique, valuable, whole human person! There is not another one in the world just like you!**

Inward Dignity and YOU!
Ppt No. 13, Lesson 2

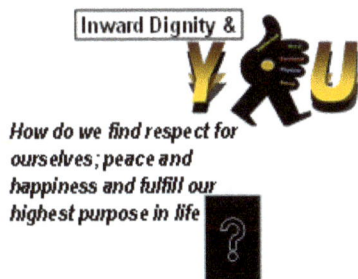

Inward Dignity & YOU

How do we find respect for ourselves; peace and happiness and fulfill our highest purpose in life?

The question is: *If we are a unique, valuable and whole person with dignity, how do we find respect for ourselves, peace and happiness and fulfill our highest purpose in life?* The earlier in life we answer this question the healthier we will be individually and in all of our relationships.

Remember we all long and desire good things. We all develop as whole persons with an intellect, moral, emotional, physical and social aspects. As we experience life and mature in our relationships socially, we develop trust based on our innate desire for connectedness and respect for our dignity as a human person.

No one wants to be used and abused. Even a young toddler knows the difference when someone intentionally trips them or when it is an accident. We all long to be respected and valued as a whole person. We long for peace and happiness.

We cannot expect the respect from others until we respect and set boundaries for ourselves. Happiness cannot be found until we have peace. Peace cannot be found until we understand our intrinsic value, innate desire for connectedness, dignity and the makeup of the whole person.

Lesson 2 Classroom Continued

The popular media equates the outward conditions, physical looks, performances, success, power and even sex with happiness. None of these will ever really satisfy the deep longing, innate desire for peace, happiness and unconditional love.

The way we define peace and love will determine how we live our lives, what we think is most important, how we treat other people, what we mean by success and quality of life, how we view human rights. . . even how we view ourselves as whole persons!

Human beings have intellectual, moral, emotional, physical and social aspects that make us who we are. It is important that while we are young, we form a personal identity that reflects the wholeness of human nature.

Question:
As a whole person with intrinsic dignity, have you found peace, happiness, meaning and purpose in your life?

Applying Extrinsic & Intrinsic Value to Relationships
Remember we are endowed with rights, and as humans we have the power to love and create other human beings. As humans, we also have the freedom to choose to use these rights and powers in our interactions with others while expressing our love and our sexuality.

On the next two powerpoints, let's see how applying extrinsic and intrinsic value to our relationships with others will affect how we express our love and sexuality toward them:

Ppt. No.14, Lesson 2

Applying Extrinsic Value to Relationships

Extrinsic: "I love you because of your looks or appearance." So in the relationship I treat you as a sexual thing or object.

or "I love you because you like my looks, and I can control your emotions." So, in the relationship I treat you as something I have conquered or my sexual trophy.

To apply **extrinsic value** to relationships is selfish and trying to get something for one's self.

Lesson 2 Classroom Continued

Applying Extrinsic Value to Relationships: "I love you because of your looks or appearance." So, in the relationship I treat you as a sexual thing or object. Or..."I love you because you like my looks, and I can control your emotions." So, in the relationship I treat you as something I have conquered or my sexual trophy. To apply extrinsic value to relationships is selfish and trying to get something for one's self. It could be manipulative and produce feelings of jealousy, distrust, irresponsibility and demanding of one's own way. Love and relationships based on extrinsic value do not last.

Question:
Are you being treated as a sexual thing or object by someone else? If so you have the "right" as a human person to protect your life and your emotions. Write your thoughts here:

Ppt. No. 15, Lesson 2

Applying Intrinsic Value to Relationships

Intrinsic:"I love you because you have value as a human being and I want to give my whole self to you. I love you because I recognize that you are a whole person and you have meaning and purpose." So in the relationship I treat you with respect and dignity. I place honor on a sexual union in a lifelong marriage and celebrate our children as a heritage of our love."
And...And..."I choose to love you with the same unconditional love that I am free to receive so others can see the example in our relationship."
To apply intrinsic value to relationships is selfless and giving of one's self to the other.

Applying Intrinsic Value to Relationships:
"I love you because you have value as a human being and I want to give my whole self to you. I love you because I recognize that you are a whole person and you have meaning and purpose."

So, in the relationship I treat you with respect and dignity. I place honor on a sexual union in a lifelong marriage and celebrate our children as a heritage of our love.

And..."I choose to love you with the same unconditional love that I am free to receive so others can see the example in our relationship." To apply intrinsic value to relationships is selfless and giving of one's self to the other. Once a marriage counselor was asked to write an article for *Bride* magazine titled, "*What Makes a Marriage Work*". He said he could sum it up in one, nine letter word, "SACRIFICE!"

Question: Are you applying intrinsic value to your relationships? If so, how will this help you in choosing to love unconditionally?

Lesson 2 Classroom Continued

The following definition of unconditional love can be useful in treating others with respect and dignity as humans and applying intrinsic value to our relationships.

Ppt. No. 16, Lesson 2

UNCONDITIONAL LOVE
is patient and kind.
It does not envy.
It does not boast.
It is not proud.
It is not rude.
It is not self-seeking.
It is not easily angered.
It keeps no record of wrongs.
Unconditional love does not delight in evil.
And it rejoices in the truth.
It always protects, always hopes and always perseveres.
Unconditional love never fails.

Question: **Remember the definition of Sexual Health is.** . . *living out one's sexuality in true freedom with integrity, purity and unconditional love. It is making healthy choices in relationships, love, and responsibility that will affect the whole person present and future and the heritage passed on to future generations.* Take a moment and write down any areas you would like to change in your life. This is personal and private so it is good to put the date, place and time on it so you can look back later and see your progress.

Let's review the five aspects of the whole person on five fingers. Show your neighbor your respect for their dignity as a whole person by giving them a high five!

Ppt. No 17, Lesson 2

As a
WHOLE
Person

YOU are
Uniquely
Different!

For the Teacher Lesson 3 Concepts

Love & Responsibility
This lesson will teach that true love requires sacrifice. We have chosen to use the *Love & Life at the Movies: Growing in Love with the Film Classics, Roman Holiday Love and Responsibility* ©Educational Guidance Institute, Inc., 2008 [35]

You will need to have the film, ***Roman Holiday***, for lessons 3 and 4. It is available for rent/purchase on YouTube, Amazon, WalMart, etc.

Note: *Each teacher may choose to present the film parts within a different time schedule.* **In order to show Roman Holiday Part One and Two during Lesson 3 and Part Three and Four during Lesson 4, class times must be based on a 90-minute schedule. For 45 min. class times, divide Lesson 3 into two class sessions and Lesson 4 into two class sessions.** *It is important to check out the video equipment etc., prior to class time. Some DVD players or computers may not have capability for scene selection, and online videos may need to buffer.*

Lesson 3 Classroom
Love & Life at the Movies: Growing in Love with the Film Classics
Roman Holiday Love & Responsibility
(used by permission from Love & Life at the Movie: Growing in Love with the Film Classics, Roman Holiday Love & Responsibility, Educational Guidance Institute ©2008)

Introduction

Today, we're going to watch the first half of a classic film. Does anyone know what a classic film is, or what comes to your mind, when you hear "classic film"? Old, black and white?…There is actually a Motion Picture Code, known as the Hays Code that was adopted on March 31st, 1930 that Hollywood agreed to follow. In order for a film to be considered a classic film, it must meet the following criteria:

General Principles

The code says that no picture shall be produced that will lower the moral standards of those who see it and that correct standards of life shall be presented.

Sexuality

The sanctity of marriage and the home shall be upheld, and pictures should not infer that low forms of sexual relationships are the accepted or common thing. It also said that adultery, while sometimes necessary for the plot, must not be justified or presented attractively and that scenes of passion should not be introduced when not essential to the plot, and must not be excessive. No lustful kissing, embraces or suggestive postures should be shown.

So, does that sound like a lot of the movies you see today? It sure doesn't to me. The other thing that classic films present could be called whole person romance. This means that all five parts of your being; intellectual, mental, physical, emotional and social are issues in attraction and generating real romance in a relationship. Classic films portray sexual relationships in marriage in a positive light and sexual relationships outside of marriage in a negative light. Current research indicates that married people tend to be happier and healthier AND experience greater sexual fulfillment in their relationships than people who cohabitate or "hook-up".

This movie will be different in that regard to other movies you may be watching. But I think you'll really enjoy this film. Before we start watching, let's go over a few facts about it.

Lesson 3 Classroom Continued

Ppt. 1, Lesson 3

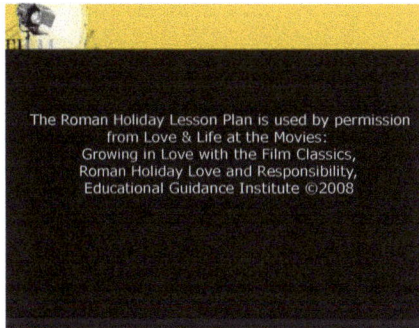

Ppt. 2, Lesson 3

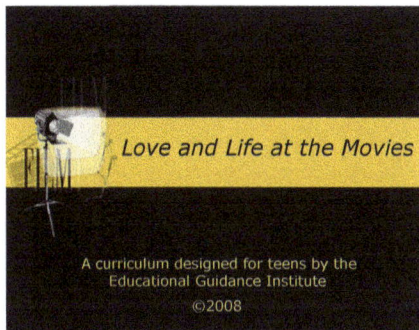

The name of the film is *Roman Holiday*.

Ppt. 3, Lesson 3

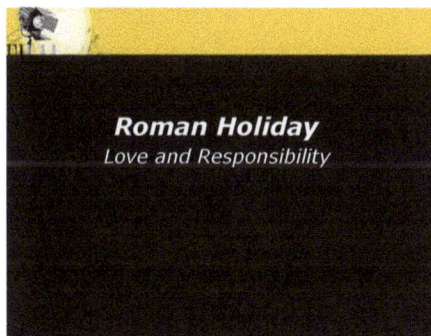

It stars Audrey Hepburn. Has anyone heard of her? It was filmed in Rome, so you'll see famous landmarks, like the Coliseum.

Ppt. 4, Lesson 3

Lesson 3 Classroom Continued

This film won three Oscars and was Audrey Hepburn's debut film.

Ppt. 5, Lesson 3

Film History and Background

Roman Holiday was nominated for seven Academy Awards (Oscars) and won three. It was also nominated for a Directors Guild of America award and won the Golden Globe Award for Best Motion Picture Actress.

Roman Holiday was the screen debut for Audrey Hepburn, and it won her an academy award for "Best Actress in a Leading Role."

Another concept about classic films is that they are worth watching again and again. Also, like I mentioned before, we will watch the entire movie. It will be broken down into 4 parts, with breaks to discuss a few key points over the course of the next 2 (or 4) class periods.

Ppt. 6, Lesson 3

Watching the Classics

Classic Films –well worth watching again and again!

The film will be viewed in its entirety.

This is a "character education" activity, where we will analyze plot and character.

Each part will have a theme. The first theme is: *"The glamorous life of wealth and fame is not always as wonderful as it appears."* Be watching for how you see this play out in the first part/segment of the movie.

Ppt. 7, Lesson 3

Part One: The Princess Escapes

Notice how the theme for this segment is reflected in the film:

The glamorous life of wealth and fame is not always as wonderful as it appears.

Lesson 3 Classroom Continued

Grab your journals (or notebook paper) and write down these key terms and definitions:
Gracious: Showing courtesy and kindness to others regardless of social standing.
Vulnerable: Without defenses to abuse or attack.
Overwhelmed: Made helpless by the burdens of your status or duties.
Self -Control: The ability to control your actions and desires by reason rather than emotion.

Ppt. 8, Lesson 3

Key Terms

- **Gracious:** Showing courtesy, charm, and kindness to others, regardless of rank or social standing.
- **Vulnerable:** Unprotected and without defenses to abuse or attack.
- **Overwhelmed:** Made helpless by the burden of one's status, office, or duties.
- **Self-control:** The ability to control one's actions and desires by one's reason rather than emotions.

ROLL THE FILM!
Film Time: 29 min.

(Show Part One of Film – The Princess Escapes - film time 29 minutes. **Part One ends at the end of the palace scene when the ambassador says, *"We must notify their majesties…")***

(Roman Holiday Discussion Questions are on the Ppt. and used by permission in the student journals, therefore, they cannot be duplicated.)

You can follow along as we discuss and answer these questions in your journals (or notebook paper).

Where did you see our keywords play out in the characters? Irving was the man who hosted the poker game.

Ppt. 9, Lesson 3

Character Traits

What character traits did you see in the following characters?

- Princess Anne
- Joe Bradley
- Irving Radovich

How do we know that Princess Anne is wealthy?

Even though, she has all that, she is still unhappy. Why?

Lesson 3 Classroom Continued

Ppt.10, Lesson 3

Discussion of Segment One

Princess Anne is obviously a wealthy celebrity. Name some of the things she has.

Why is Anne unhappy even though she has all of these things?

What is significant about the scene when Anne asks "is the elevator"? (It shows how vulnerable she is and that she has no idea what has just happened.)

Ppt. 11, Lesson 3

Discussion of Segment One

"Is this the elevator?" – Anne
"It's my room." – Joe Bradley

What is significant in the scene in which Joe takes Anne to his apartment for the night?

Let's see what happens next in our film. The theme for Part Two is *"exercising self-control with members of the opposite sex is necessary for trust in a relationship".* Keep that theme in mind as we watch this next segment.

Ppt. 12, Lesson 3

Part Two: Joe Bradley Finds a Story

Notice how the theme for this segment is reflected in the film:

Exercising self-control with members of the opposite sex is necessary for trust in a relationship.

Before we start part two, grab your journals (or notebook paper) and jot down these definitions.

Modesty: The virtue of keeping private that which should be private (body, language etc.)

Opportunist: Someone who take advantage of a situation to achieve their goals without considering how it might hurt others.

Ppt. 13, Lesson 3

(Show Part Two of the film. Begin approximately 1 ½ min. before end of Scene 6 film time 32 minutes. **Segment two ends as Princess Anne leaves the barber shop.)**

Our key words were modesty and opportunist. Which traits did you see in each of the characters?

Ppt. 14, Lesson 3

How does Anne know that she can trust Joe Bradley?

Lesson 3 Classroom Continued

Ppt. 15, Lesson 3

Character Concept

Anne is alarmed, as any girl would be, to find herself in a strange man's apartment after having spent the night there. Anne realizes, however, that Joe took her off the street and gave her a place to stay without taking advantage of her. Because he exercised self-control when she was most vulnerable, she knows she can trust him.

In the first part of the film we really liked Joe Bradley. He was gracious and used self-control. How do we now see that he is a complex character?

Ppt. 16, Lesson 3

Discussion of Segment Two

How is Joe Bradley a complex character? What virtues and flaws do we see in him?

As we discussed earlier, Princess Anne trusts Joe Bradley. This scene shows specifically why she feels that she can trust him.

Ppt. 17, Lesson 3

Discussion of Segment Two

"Have I been here all night . . . alone?" – Anne
"If you don't count me, yes." – Joe
"So I've spent the night here – with you." - Anne
"Oh, well, now, I – I don't know if I'd use those words exac
but er, from a certain angle, yes." – Joe
Why does Anne feel she can trust

Joe Bradley?

Do you like the film so far? Next week, we'll watch the rest of the film. Be sure to bring your journals (or paper to write down your answers) and be working on memorizing the definition of Sexual Health!

For the Teacher Lesson 4 Concepts
Love & Responsibility cont.

This lesson will teach that true love requires sacrifice using the *Love & Life at the Movies Growing in Love with the Film Classics Roman Holiday Love and Responsibility* ©Educational Guidance Institute, Inc., 2008 [36]

You will need to have the film, ***Roman Holiday***, for lessons 3 and 4. It is available for rent/purchase on YouTube, Amazon, WalMart, etc.

Note: Each teacher may choose to present the film segments within a different time schedule.
In order to show Roman Holiday Part One and Two during Lesson 3 and Part Three and Four during Lesson 4 class times must be based on a 90-minute schedule. For 45 min. class times, divide Lesson 3 into two class sessions and Lesson 4 into two class sessions. *It is important to check out the video equipment etc, prior to class time. Some DVD players or computers may not have capability for scene selection, and online videos may need to buffer.*

Lesson 4 Classroom
Love & Life at the Movies Growing in Love with the Film Classics
Roman Holiday Love & Responsibility

Introduction

Today we will wrap up our movie. You can get your journals (or paper) out, as you will need them later.

Let's review for anyone who might not have been here or remember what's happening. (*Give students the opportunity to recap what happened in parts one and two of the film.*)

We have a princess, Anne, who was overwhelmed with her situation. She was given a shot by her doctor that made her tired and seem drugged or intoxicated. She escaped from the palace and was in a very vulnerable state and fell asleep on a bench. A reporter, Joe Bradley, found her and let her sleep at his apartment for the night. He didn't know who she was. The next day, he found out she was a princess and decided he was going to use her to get a story. She is loving being able to make decisions for herself, and when we ended part two, she was just leaving the barber shop and had got her hair cut short.

Now that everyone is caught up, let's see what the theme is for Part Three of the movie. *"Honesty is an essential element in true friendship."* Remember to be looking for this to play out as you watch the film.

Ppt. 1, Lesson 4

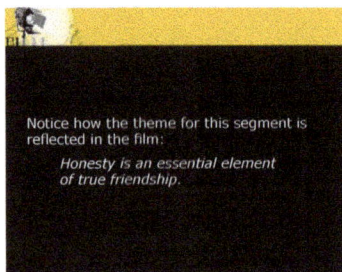

In your journals (or notebook paper) write the definitions for these two words:

Collaborator: One who cooperates with another in a joint effort (often in a shady deal or treachery).

Deceitful: Intending to trick or mislead someone.

Lesson 4 Classroom Continued

Ppt. 2, Lesson 4

Key Terms

Collaborator: One who cooperates with another in a joint effort (often in a shady deal or treachery).

Deceitful: Intending to trick or mislead someone.

ROLL THE FILM!
Film Time: 30 min.

(Show Part Three of Film – A Day in Rome, Scene 11 film time 30 minutes. **Segment three ends as Princess Anne and Joe Bradley kiss by the car.)**

Let's look at our characters again to see what traits we saw this time. Remember our key terms were collaborator and deceitful.

Ppt. 3, Lesson 4

Character Traits

What character traits did you see in the following characters during this segment?

Princess Anne
Joe Bradley Irving
Radovich

As they ended with a kiss, it's becoming clear that Anne is falling in love with Joe Bradley. This scene is the first time we get that notion. Looking at this scene, why does Anne fall in love with Joe?

Ppt. 4, Lesson 4

Discussion of Segment Three

"You spent the whole day doing things I've always wanted to. Why?" – Anne
"I don't know. Seemed the thing to do." – Joe
"I never heard of anybody so kind." – Anne

Why does Anne fall in love with Joe?

Did you notice when they were talking on the barge and there was a moment that he couldn't look her in the eyes, but instead he looked down? He knows that he is being deceitful, and taking advantage of the Princess by creating a story on her.

Lesson 4 Classroom Continued

Ppt. 5, Lesson 4

Discussion of Segment Three

When does Joe begin to realize that his character is lacking in some respects? Why does he feel bad about this?

We're almost done with the film. In Part Four, we'll see that True love requires doing one's duty and acting responsibly, which usually involves making sacrifices.

Ppt. 6, Lesson 4

Part Four: A Bittersweet Parting

Notice how the theme for this segment is reflected in the film:

True love requires doing one's duty and acting responsibly, which usually involves making sacrifices.

Get your journals (or notebook paper) out one more time and write down our last keywords for the film.

Sacrifice: Giving up someone or something that is dear to us for the sake of something that is of greater value.

Responsibility: Trustworthiness; faithfulness to one's duties.

Ppt. 7, Lesson 4

Key Terms

Sacrifice: Giving up someone or something that is dear to us for the sake of someone or something that is of greater value.

Responsibility: Trustworthiness; faithfulness to one's duties.

ROLL THE FILM!
Film Time: 26 min.

(Show Part Four of Film – A Bittersweet Parting, Scene 16 film time 26 minutes. Film ends.)

Lesson 4 Classroom Continued

What did you think of the film? Some of you are disappointed that they didn't end up together. Some of you have said that you thought it would end similarly to this way.

Let's discuss what traits we saw in each of these characters. What did you think of Irving for most of the film? We saw that he was a collaborator and deceitful among other things. But, at the end, did you notice what he did? He pulled out the lighter with which he was taking pictures when Princess Anne walked in the room. Then he gave her the pictures.

Ppt. 8, Lesson 4

> **Character Traits**
>
> What character traits did you see in the following characters during this segment?
>
> Princess Anne
> Joe Bradley Irving
> Radovich

Joe makes a sacrifice because he loves Princess Anne. They both also know the responsibility that Anne has as Princess.

Ppt. 9, Lesson 4

> **Discussion of Segment Four**
>
> How does Joe's decision to let Anne go back to the palace reflect his love for her?

What is Joe saying here? He's saying that because he cares for the Princess, he will not share the story. He values her and their relationship.

Ppt. 10, Lesson 4

> **Discussion of Segment Four**
>
> "And what, in the opinion of Your Highness, is the outlook for friendship among nations?" – Reporter
> "I have every faith in it . . . As I have faith in relations between people." – Princess Anne
> "May I say, speaking for my own press service: we believe your highness's faith will not be unjustified." – Joe Bradley
>
> What do these quotes say about the trust Anne has in Joe and also about the love Joe has for Anne?

Lesson 4 Classroom Continued

We know that Joe could have really used the money he could have been paid to write this story. But because he loved her, he made a sacrifice.

This is not the fairy tale ending we're used to seeing in most movies, is it? But, in a way, it's even better. Even though they didn't end up together, they both left the relationship "whole". We've talked a lot about the whole person in these lessons, and neither of them gave the other anything they can't get back. Remember Dan and Jan – the heart activity in Lesson 1? They left a piece of each other on each other's hearts because they had sex, not to mention all the bonding they shared that scientifically takes time to heal. Joe and Princess Anne never crossed that line. So, although it will take some time for them to move on, they are both still whole, will be able to move on and find true love.

Ppt. 11, Lesson 4

> **Program Application**
>
> At the end of the movie, we see Joe give up Anne (and forfeit his opportunity to make $5,000 by not printing the story) so that she can do her duty. Explain how this sacrifice will allow them both to be happy.

(After the conclusion of the film and all of its discussion questions, please continue with the following:)

Question: Do you dream of falling in love and possibly getting married someday? If so, write down how you will meet, what characteristics your dream lover will have, their attitudes and behaviors; and how you will fall in love. Also, add any plans you may have to get married and have children. Tell what the relationship will involve and begin to live your dream. It is possible!

Remember the definition of Sexual Health is.... *living out one's sexuality in true freedom with integrity, purity and unconditional love. It is making healthy choices in relationships, love, and responsibility that will affect the whole person present and future and the heritage passed on to future generations.*

Question: If you are currently involved in a relationship, do you see it producing your dream results? If not, why do we accept less than the best for ourselves?

For the Teacher Lesson 5 Concepts

Are You Dying to Have Sex or Saving Sex for One Monogamous Bond?
A human person has the ability to reason and make choices. Our bodies can be trained to live with sexual health. In this lesson the difference between love and lust is explored along with the medical facts of sexually transmitted diseases/STD's/STI's. The majority of this lesson is based on students exploring the consequences of STD's and the results of having sex outside of marriage or one monogamous bond. Since contraceptives do not always provide protection against STDs, have negative physical consequences of artificial hormones on the body and the negative emotional consequences on relationships, this curriculum explains but does not promote their use. However, it will be explained that there are other medical reasons for their use. Students will be presented information concerning family planning that has healthier results than artificial contraceptives. Students will understand the current epidemic of STDs/STIs. Students are encouraged to examine the data and to consider the long-term outcomes of the potential risks of multiple sexual partners as compared to a monogamous relationship as the safest way to avoid STDs/STIs.

Objectives:
1) Students will be able to identify the increase in sexual activity and the negative habits in relationships through the use of contraceptives reducing love to lust with at least 75% participation from the class.
2) With at least 90% participation and through discussion of the STD activity, students will be able to compare and contrast the risks of contracting multiple STDs and the negative consequences of multiple sexual partners to the benefits of one monogamous relationship with unconditional love.
3) At the end of the lesson, students will be able to describe the difference between bacterial, viral, and parasitic STDs and the negative physical and emotional consequences to their sexual health. Students will complete a Pre/Post test with 90% accuracy and participation.
4) Practical Ways to Handle Sexual Temptation can be learned.

Lesson Plan

Permission is given by the authors to insert applicable substitutes for video clip/s, handouts, or slides based on current stats/population/culture maintaining the meaning and values of the original content.

Activity: STD's are a Sticky Business (You will need a piece of chewing gum for each student.)

Journal Pages

Handouts: Pre/Post STD Test, Appendix, Lesson 5
Sexual Exposure Chart, Appendix, Lesson 5

Lecture & Discussion

PowerPoints (Ppts): (1) Concepts of Truth's Definition of Sexual Health (2) Choices, Choices (3) Planning My Future (4) Actions Do Speak Louder Than Words (5) Don't Advertise What You Don't Want To Sell (6) Love vs. Lust (7) Female Fertility Cycle

YouTube clip Pornography- Russell Brand

Video/slides on STD's (Allow approx. 25-30 min.)

Lesson 5 Classroom
Are You Dying to Have Sex or Saving Sex for One Monogamous Bond?

Introduction:
How many of you want to get married or save sex for one monogamous bond? We can find our prince or princess. (Show first slide of wedding pic.) People have the ability to reason and make choices. Choices produce healthy or unhealthy consequences. Our bodies can be trained to live with sexual health.

We know sexual health is...*living out one's sexuality in true freedom with integrity, purity and unconditional love. It is making healthy choices in relationships, love, and responsibility that will affect the whole person present and future and the heritage passed on to future generations.* So, let's review and say it together:

Ppt 1, Lesson 5

(Concepts of Truth's Definition)
SexualHealth is.........
living out one's sexuality in true freedom with integrity, purity and unconditional love.

It is making healthy choices in relationships, love and responsibility that will affect the whole person present and future and the heritage passed on to future generations.

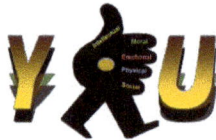

Question:
Do you feel like you are living out your sexuality in true freedom?   YES   NO
Explain:

We sometimes make decisions that are unhealthy because we don't have direction. In some cases, bad things happened when we were younger, and were unable to control the situation. If this has happened to you, it is not your fault. For those things over which we had no control, there is help to heal the pain. If you need help, please call our confidential helpline at **1.866.482.LIFE.**

For those things we can control, it is good to recognize how important our decisions are today. Remember, you can choose relationships that reflect unconditional love and pass on a healthy heritage for your children.

Lesson 5 Classroom Continued

Question:

What choices are you making?

Ppt No. 2, Lesson 5

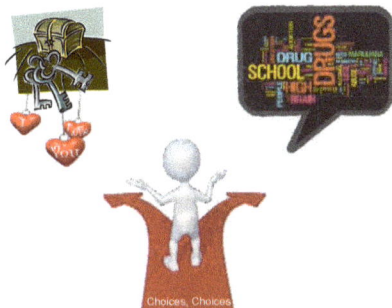

Remember our choices affect our whole person. They affect us intellectually, morally, emotionally, physically and socially. Look at the next power ppt. revealing some good consequences based on whether one chooses to save sex for one monogamous partner. Our choices concerning our attitudes and behaviors about sex can be healthy and the consequences can be good!

Ppt No. 3, Lesson 5

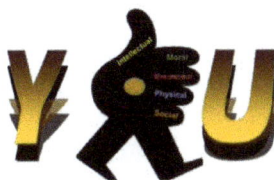

Our Choices Affect The Whole Person

Good consequences can be yours if you save sex for one monogamous bond.

Intellectual
Graduate
High Self-Esteem

Emotional
No Regret
Happy
Have a Life
Confident
Stable
Without Hurt

Moral
Right Thinking
Peace
Connected

Physical
Future Children
Healthy Relationships
Sexual Health
Marriage

Social
Financially Secure
Good Reputation
Respect Boyfriend/girlfriend
Married with Unitive Intimacy

Lesson 5 Classroom Continued

Our behaviors say a lot about who we are, how we view ourselves, what we think of others and what we believe.

Ppt. No. 4, Lesson 5

Sometimes we say one thing, but our body language and behaviors are saying something else and we send the wrong message.

For example, if a girl says she wants to remain pure but she wears clothes that make her look like a hooker; or if a guy says he wants to be pure but is bragging about his one night stands. Do you agree that actions speak louder than words?

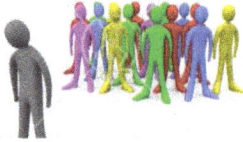

Ppt. No. 5, Lesson 5

Question: Don't advertise what you don't want to sell.
Actions speak louder than words. Do your actions or behaviors tell the truth about who you really are?

Remember, sexual health is living out your sexuality (that is who you are) in true freedom, with integrity, purity, and unconditional love.

Question:
How would you change your behavior to portray a better picture of who you really are?

Lesson 5 Classroom Continued

Lust or Love?

If sexual health includes true freedom, integrity, purity, and unconditional love, then sex is good and pure and right. If sex is good, why do people accept being used as a tool, hooking up, or being a friend with benefits?

People who do not know how to live with sexual health experience second rate sex in relationships outside of marriage or one monogamous bond. This causes pain and brokenness and people get hurt. *(Optional - Show YouTube clip Pornography – Russell Brand instead of reading next two paragraphs. It is included in the digital curriculum and inserted in the powerpoint slides before the slide on lust or love.)*

For some men and women, fantasy or illicit relationships are what drive them sexually. Because of this, they may be drawn to the wrong kinds of people and find it difficult to stop risky behavior. They could become hypersensitized to pictures and or objects desensitizing themselves to human sexual relationships.

Masturbation and pornography are behaviors where young people think, "no one is getting hurt," only to find out years later they wish they had been right. A person who develops a porn or masturbation lifestyle at a young age will, more often than not, carry those habits into the marriage and cause difficulty in the relationship.

Now is a good time to start making some decisions about how you will let yourself be treated. Remember you can start practicing secondary virginity that we discussed in Lesson 1.

Question:
Have you created habits or relationship behaviors that are unhealthy?

Lesson 1 explained that real love can only come through making a total gift of self in the commitment to one monogamous partner and hopefully for a lifetime.

Love involves a sacrifice of self, respecting the other person, not using them and surrendering yourself to an unconditional love that can be modeled in your relationship as an example to others.

Lesson 5 Classroom Continued

Hookups or friends with benefits are based on lust, extrinsic value, are temporary and reduces the person to an object to be used. Remember the average high school relationship after having sex is only 3 weeks long. Compare the characteristics of lust and love in the following powerpoint list as we read them together:

Ppt No. 6, Lesson 5
Lust vs. Love

Lust
- Temporary
- Based on fantasy
- Shallow
- Selfish
- Sudden
- Can't wait to get
- Focuses on external looks
- Full of emotion

Love
- Enduring
- Based on reality
- Deep
- Unselfish
- Gradual
- Can't wait to give
- Focuses on internal character
- Full of devotion

Question:
Do you feel used and abused in your relationship/s?

Contraceptives (Birth Control)
Most people will agree since contraceptives are more available sexual activity has increased among teens. The popular media reported on, and even promoted, casual acceptance of the pill as early as 1963.

The pill allowed people to separate sex from pregnancy. However, one's moral conscience is still affected. STDs, their negative outcomes, and abortion has risen in numbers since the sexual revolution of the 60's. Research tells us that birth control does not always protect against STDs. Also, many teens don't use contraceptives consistently. Some females have said if they got pregnant without taking the pill they felt less guilty. The moral conscience of the whole person is affected.

Birth control pills were first introduced as helpful to women for reproductive freedom, but in fact, some have caused many women to have health problems.

Lesson 5 Classroom Continued

Please check out some of the resources we list in your journal such as the online brochure, *If it's not OK for him to take steroids. . .why is it OK for her?* by Breast Cancer Prevention Institute at www.bcpinstitute.org[37] You will find that because more younger women are taking the pill, many of them are getting breast cancer at a younger age.

Many of the pills act like an abortifacient *(a substance that induces abortion)* preventing implantation of the fertilized egg.

If you are on the pill because of medical problems, please consult with your doctor. Many people are unaware of the serious side effects of using the pill and other artificial hormones. You might want to discuss with your doctor how these artificial hormones can affect your body.

There are healthier alternatives such as **natural family planning methods**[38] that have no side effects and are based on a female understanding the days she is fertile. These natural methods have been proven to be as effective as the pill. Couples have reported a greater respect and intimacy in their relationships.

The following ppt shows a fertility chart used by natural family planning methods. Also check out the FEMM Foundation app, which helps women track their body changes.

Ppt No. 7, Lesson 5

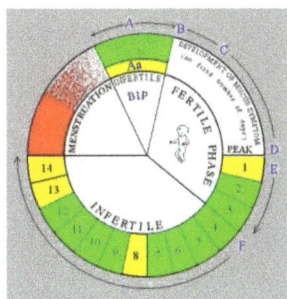

Question:
What is your opinion about contraceptives?

Lesson 5 Classroom Continued

Question:
How does the availability of contraceptives contribute to increased sexual activity outside of marriage?

Activity: STD's are Sticky Business - (You will need a piece of gum for each student who participates.)

Please take a piece of gum and begin to chew it, but make sure you save your wrapper. (Allow a short time for students to enjoy the gum.) Now, please put your gum back in the wrapper and place it in the collection basket. (Teacher mixes up the pieces of gum and offers them back to the students.) Now, you may find your piece of gum and chew it again. (The responses will probably be "Yuck", "no way", etc.)

Most of you do not want to attempt to find your gum because you are afraid that you will get someone else's, correct? I don't think anyone wants to put gum in his or her mouth knowing it has been in someone else's mouth, correct? Then why would a person have sex with more than one partner if he or she weren't absolutely sure that person had never had sex with anyone else? Research tells us that sexually transmitted diseases are passed from person to person in bodily fluids or by body contact. If this activity is symbolic of having sex with more than one partner and you choose to take the gum back again, would anyone be disease free?

Just like refusing to take the gum back, everyone has a choice to save sex for one monogamous partner. Let's look at a handout and see how a person's risk of contracting a sexually transmitted disease is exponentially multiplied when having multiple sex partners.

Handout: *Sexual Exposure Chart, Appendix, Lesson 5* [39]
(Note: 45-minute class time end here.)

(Note: 45-minute class time begin here.)

Handout: STD Pre/Post Test[40]

Take a few minutes and answer the questions on the Pre/Post test the best you can. Then listen as we watch the slides/video and you can check the answers. The test is not graded. It is simply to see how much you know about STDs before we view the information. What does STD stand for? (*Sexually Transmitted Disease*) or sometimes you may hear them called STIs.

The following slides/video will cover some of the most common bacterial, viral and parasitic sexually transmitted diseases.[41]

Show the Slides/Video[42](Allow 25-**30** min. Take time to discuss briefly.)

(Give students time to answer the *STD Pre/Post Test* questions and check answers using Answer Key in Teacher's manual)

Question:
What new information did you learn about STDs today? How will this new information affect your future sexual decisions and/or those of your current and future relationships?

Question:
Do you think a person might lie to a potential sexual partner about their past? Would this affect your decision to engage in sex with someone if you could not be sure of their sexual history?

(**Note**: Because of the time needed in this lesson the last journal page should be assigned for students to read outside of class.)

Lesson 5 Classroom Continued

Practical Ways to Handle Sexual Temptation

1. **Be absolutely convinced and fully aware of the consequences** if you fail to limit your sexual partners to one mutually monogamous relationship for life.

2. **Write out your decision about sex**. Put a reminder of this decision someplace where you will see it and remember this commitment you've made to yourself and your future.

3. **Develop Self-Esteem - believe in yourself**! If you realize you are a person of worth, with opinions of great value, you can develop a confidence in what you think and how you act.

4. **Practice Assertiveness.** Everyone has the right to make decisions concerning his or her body, especially when one's health is at stake. It is also important to realize that the mind and heart can control the body's urges!

5. **Communicate your boundaries to your date**. Make sure you talk frequently about these important issues.

6. **Don't date individuals who are disrespectful of you and your boundaries**. If you're being pressured, step back and reevaluate this relationship.

7. **Plan your dates**. Make sure you have packed your date with fun and positive things to help you get to know each other better. Too much time with nothing planned can get you into trouble.

8. **Avoid alcohol and drugs!** Alcohol and drugs deaden the mind and the ability to think and decide clearly. You could come away from your "good time" with a great deal more than you bargained for!

9. **Limit the amount of and time spent on physical involvement**. Don't spend excessive amounts of time "making out" or "exploring". This will only lead to frustration and regret. Keep it short and sweet!

10. **Find a good friend with the same resolve about sex**. Make sure you have someone you can talk to. The two of you will be able to help each other through the "pressure" times and come away with a valuable and strong relationship.[43]

Lesson 5 Classroom Continued

Resources

FEMM Foundation App - Download free app to track body changes and learn more about your body as a woman.

Books:
Kissed the Girls and Made them Cry, Why Women Lose When they Give In ©2002
Lisa Bevere Thomas Nelson, Nashville, TN

Date or Soul Mate? How to Know if Someone is Worth Pursuing in Two Dates or Less ©2002
Neil Clark Warren, PH. D. Thomas Nelson, Nashville, TN

Website for Teens:
www.decisionschoicesandoptions.org

Online Brochures on Contraceptives:

www.heritagehouse76.com
Ella
RU-486
Morning After Pill, Plan B
Depo-Provera
IUD
Condoms
Natural Family Planning

Online Brochure:
If it's not OK for him to take steroids...why is it OK for her? Breast Cancer Prevention Institute www.bcpinstitute.org

The Billings Ovulation Method™ is used by millions of women around the world. It was developed by Drs. John and Evelyn Billings, validated by eminent international scientists and verified as extremely effective by the World Health Organization. By identifying the natural signals of fertility this Method can be used to become pregnant or avoid pregnancy and to safeguard reproductive health. www.billingslife.org

For the Teacher Lesson 6 Concepts

Future Sexual Health Plans - Sex & You

Reviewing the physical and emotional cost of sex outside of the bonds of a permanent, monogamous relationship will help students understand the significance of living with sexual health in true freedom, integrity, purity and unconditional love. When students begin to grasp the value of sexual health, their lives can change positively impacting their future choices, relationships and academic goals. In the video, *The High Cost of Free Love*,[44] Pam Stenzel stresses the importance and value of sexual health in an uplifting, dramatic way. Also, allowing students to evaluate this program is important. The evaluation gives them a voice to agree or disagree to remain pure until marriage or sex with one monogamous partner, and also gives them the opportunity to recommend the program to others. Students receive a business size commitment card that can serve them in the future as a contract to live out the values and concepts of sexual health. Teachers have the opportunity to reward those who learn the definition of sexual health and also remind the students about the services of the local pregnancy center.

Objectives

1) Students will apply the knowledge they have learned by writing the definition of sexual health with 100% accuracy with at least 90% of students participating. Those who are successful will be rewarded by their name going into a drawing for free movie tickets.

2) Students will be able to describe how the *Concepts of Sexual Health Sex & You* program has helped them understand the definition of sexual health with 75% of students participating.

3) Students will give feedback through evaluating the program concerning their plans to apply the benefits of living out the definition of sexual health and recommending the program to others with 90% student participation.

Lesson Plan

Permission is given by the authors to insert applicable substitutes for video clip/s, handouts, or slides based on current stats/population/culture maintaining the meaning and values of the original content.

Activity: Drawing for Movie Tickets

Handouts: Student's Evaluation of the Program (Appendix, Lesson 6), SH Commitment Cards (may be ordered from Concepts of Truth, Inc. 1-870-238-4329)

Journal Pages

Lecture & Discussion

PowerPoint (Ppt): (1) Sexual Health Is . . .

Video: *The High Cost of Free Love* DVD, (www.pamstenzel.com 2012)[45]

Lesson 6 Classroom
Future Sexual Health Plans - Sex & You

Introduction
Today is the wrap up and the summary of the entire *Concepts of Sexual Health Sex & You!* program.

In the last five weeks, (45 min classes would be 11 weeks) hopefully you have learned the definition of sexual health and that living out that definition will help you in all aspects of your whole person - intellectual, moral, emotional, physical, and social.

Having sex outside of marriage or one monogamous bond increases your risk of not only pregnancy and STD's, but also all kinds of other relationship problems.

You have been taught the development and intrinsic dignity value of a human person and have had the opportunity to explore how your choices affect your future and your children's future.

You have the right to life, liberty and the security of person. Sex was created for procreation, bonding, completeness, unitive intimacy, and yes, it is pleasurable! It is healthier to save sex for marriage or one monogamous bond.

The video today will reinforce these concepts and challenge you to live out the concepts of sexual health as a whole person in order to positively influence your future choices, relationships and academic goals.

Video
Show video *The High Cost of Free Love* by Pam Stenzel DVD, www.pamstenzel.com (2012) [46] (60 min.)

(Note: 45-minute class time, start video here and play through first segment of video approx. 35 min. long. Begin with second section the next week.)

Definition of Sexual Health
Please use the evaluation form to write the definition of Sexual Health to best of your memory. Even if you think you only know part of it, you may know more than others in the class.

Lesson 6 Classroom Continued

We will draw for movie tickets (or other prizes). The person who gets the definition the closest will win. Please turn in the evaluation after you are finished so we can tally the winners of the definition. Anyone getting the definition correct will be in the drawing.

Handout: Evaluation Form, Appendix, Lesson 6
Your input on the evaluation form will be helpful for us in many ways. Rating the program for us allows us to have feedback on the program's effectiveness. The other questions are pertinent and will be used to make program improvements.

You may remain anonymous, but please indicate if you are male or female in the top right corner of the page. You do not have to put your entire name on the evaluation, just your first name and last initial so we can sort it for the drawing.

Again, your input is important to us. Thank you for being honest with your answers. Also, in future years, if you are still committed to saving sex for marriage or one monogamous partner, please let us know. It will be exciting to see how many will stay committed to living out your sexuality with integrity, purity and unconditional love.

Let's see how many got all of the following definition correct.

(Ppt. 1, Lesson 6)

(Concepts of Truth's Definition)
Sexual Health is.........

living out one's sexuality in true freedom with integrity, purity and unconditional love.

It is making healthy choices in relationships, love and responsibility that will affect the whole person present and future and the heritage passed on to future generations.

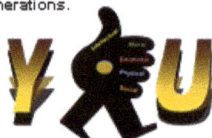

Handout: SH Commitment Cards

The SH commitment card has a place for your signature on the back if you will commit to living out the definition of sexual health. This will be a keepsake for you and also the card can be a daily reminder of your promise.

A contact phone number and web information is listed on the card. We would love for you to keep in touch with us or come by our office anytime.

Lesson 6 Classroom Continued

Question:
Remember your journals (or what you have written on paper) will be not only a keepsake from this class, but a tool to help you in the future when making decisions about your sexual health. Sexual Health is not just a one-time decision and isn't just for teens. Sexual health affects our relationships and marriage and involves a lifetime of living out our sexuality in true freedom, integrity, purity, unconditional love and passing on a heritage of life and love to the next generation. When we do so, future generations will have even better relationships than we have today. List your plans for your future academic goals, relationships, love, and responsibility.

Question:
Do you agree that having sex without the bonds of one monogamous partner has a price tag?

Question:
Explain how the *Concepts of Sexual Health Sex & You!* program has helped you understand the above statement.

Question:
HOPE AND HEALING!
Are you hurting in relationships or from past sexual decisions?
Getting help is important and there is hope for healing! Your parents, your teachers, your counselors and we can help you. The most important thing is to choose to deal and heal with any hurt in current relationships or the past before it affects your future in a negative way. We learn from our mistakes and a human person has the ability to reason and make choices. Please, choose Sexual Health! It affects **YOU** - the **WHOLE PERSON!!**

Question:
Write your thoughts here:

Closing
In closing, we thank you for participating and being attentive. We want to encourage you to never forget what you have learned and to always strive to live out the definition of sexual health.

Also, please tell someone else about what you have learned in these lessons. Remember, there is no one else in the world just like you. You are a whole person and you are valuable!

Let's see who won the movie tickets!

APPENDIX

PLANNING THE FUTURE CHECKLIST

Check the goals you want to complete in your future.

1. ____ Go to College, Trade School
2. ____ Be physically fit, strong and healthy
3. ____ Be financially stable
4. ____ Have a job (career) I love
5. ____ Get married
6. ____ Travel the world
7. ____ Have good friends
8. ____ Help others
9. ____ Have a family
10. ____ Be content
11. ____ Have a nice home
12. ____ Have security

Check the goals you want your children (or will want for your children) to complete in their future.

1. ____ Want my children to be happy
2. ____ Have a loving spouse, be loved
3. ____ Have a good job
4. ____ Be financially well off
5. ____ Be healthy
6. ____ Be comfortable
7. ____ Have nice things
8. ____ Go to school
9. ____ Safe from harm
10. ____ Enjoy being with family
11. ____ Lots of good friends
12. ____ Morally & spiritually healthy

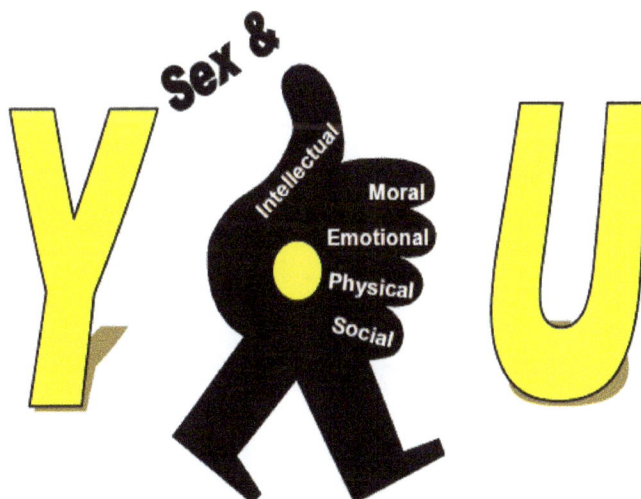

Concepts of Sexual Health

Concepts of Truth, Inc ©2010   Appendix Lesson 1

Secondary Virginity

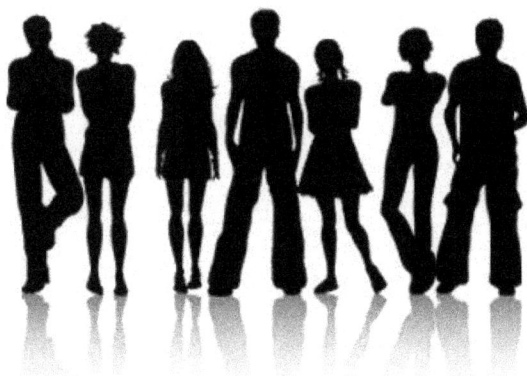

Secondary virginity is a concept, an idea that works. If you have lost your virginity by having sexual intercourse your physical virginity is lost, true fact. However, you can start today by making a decision to abstain from sexual activity until marriage or until having sex with one monogamous partner for the rest of your life. Secondary Virginity is an idea, an attitude, a frame of mind that is expressed in the way you look at yourself and others. It is a decision to allow your body time to heal from past habits and to heal emotional wounds. Secondary Virginity will allow your body time to repair bonding hormones. It is an opportunity to start fresh in a commitment to live free and renew your mind and body prior to a future commitment to have sex with one monogamous partner for the rest of your life hopefully in the bonds of marriage.

Start over today by:

- Making a firm commitment to save sex from now til marriage. YOU CAN DO IT!
- Avoid people, places, things and situations that weaken your self-control.
- Sometimes the healthiest thing we can do is avoid people who tempt us.
- Avoid intense hugging, passionate kissing and anything else that leads to lustful thoughts and behavior. Anything beyond a brief, simple kiss can quickly become dangerous.
- Find non-physical ways to show your love and appreciation.

Teen quotes:

"Just because I made a mistake doesn't mean I have to keep on making the same mistakes."
"I didn't like being used."
"I'm going to wait because it's the best for me and for my future children."

Fetal Development Test

1. The baby's first cell division occurs during
    a. first month
    b. first week
    c. first 24 hours
    d. first hour

2. In _____days the baby's heart chamber is developing.
    a. 25
    b. 10
    c. 2
    d. 32

3. The embryo's heart beats
    a. slower than the mother's
    b. twice as fast as mother's
    c. once a day
    d. every 24 hours

4. At _____weeks male or female reproductive organs are visible.
    a. 10
    b. 15
    c. 12
    d. 24

5. At 9 weeks the baby looks like a little human being and is called a/an
    a. embryo
    b. oocyte
    c. fetus
    d. none of these

6. 60,000 miles of _____bring nutrients to the baby inside the mother's womb.
    a. track
    b. arteries
    c. veins
    d. vessels

Fetal Development Test Pg. 2

7. _____ and _____ are present at 32 days.
   a. hair and finger nails
   b. arms and legs
   c. eyes and ears
   d. none of these

8. The title of this video is
   a. A Miracle
   b. First Nine Months
   c. From Conception to Birth
   d. Instruction Sets

9. What inseminates the oocyte?
   a. water
   b. egg
   c. sperm
   d. all of these

10. How does the mathematician describe his response to life in the womb?
    a. An amazement
    b. A marvel
    c. A confusion
    d. none of these

Fetal Development Test Answer Key

1. C
2. A
3. B
4. C
5. C
6. D
7. B
8. C
9. C
10. B

SEXUAL EXPOSURE CHART

(if every person has only the same number of partners as you)

Number of Sexual Partners		Number of People Exposed to
1		1
2		3
3		7
4		15
5		31
6		63
7		127
8		255
9		511
10		1023
11		2047
12		4095

STD Slides/Video Pre/Post Test

1. A person can become infected with Chlamydia through _____.
    a. sexual intercourse
    b. oral sex
    c. anal sex
    d. childbirth
    e. all of the above

2. Do people infected with Chlamydia always know it?
    Yes   No

3. What can happen to me if I have Chlamydia?
    a. Infertility
    b. Chronic pelvic pain
    c. Ectopic pregnancy
    d. PID
    e. All of the above

4. All STD's can be cured.
    True   False

5. PID only affects women.
    True   False

6. A person ALWAYS has symptoms with Gonorrhea.
    True   False

7. Syphilis can be seen on the _____.
    a. lips & mouth
    b. anus
    c. rectum
    d. vagina
    e. all of the above

8. Gonorrhea can be spread to the throat by oral sexual contact.
   True   False

9. Once a person is infected with Herpes, he/she will be infected for life.
   True   False

10. People who have NO signs or symptoms may transmit herpes.
    True   False

11. HPV is commonly known as Genital Warts.
    True   False

12. Three kinds of STD'S are
    a. Viral, Penile, Anal
    b. Bacterial, Viral, Parasitic
    c. Chronic, Lifelong, Incurable
    d. None of the above

13. HIV can be passed on through touching, hugging, kissing or other
    casual contact.
    True   False

14. There is no cure for HIV/AIDS.
    True   False

15. Which of the following STD'S/STI'S are caused by a parasite?
    a. Scabies
    b. HPV
    c. Pubic Lice
    d. Both a & c

STD Slides/Video Test Answer Key

1. E
2. No
3. E
4. False
5. True
6. False
7. E
8. True
9. True
10. True
11. True
12. B
13. False
14. True
15. D

Date_____

Name of School_____

Please circle M for male or F for female   M   F

Class Period_____

Concepts of Sexual Health Sex & You! Evaluation Sheet

(Please write the definition of Sexual Health as presented in the program)

Sexual Health is ....

Rate the *Concepts of Sexual Health Sex & You!* Program - Please rate how the program was or was not beneficial to you. Please take the time to give us your rating on the following questions. Put an X in the box under your choices. Thanks and have a healthy life.

Place an X under 1 item only for each statement.	Agree	Disagree	Undecided
1. I plan to stay pure, save sex until marriage or practice secondary virginity based on what I learned from *Concepts of Sexual Health Sex & You!*			
2. After completing *Concepts of Sexual Health Sex & You!*, I would recommend the program to others.			
3. I understand more about my sexual health as a whole person because of the *Concepts of Sexual Health Sex & You!* program.			

Please tell us something that you learned from *Concepts of Sexual Health Sex & You!*

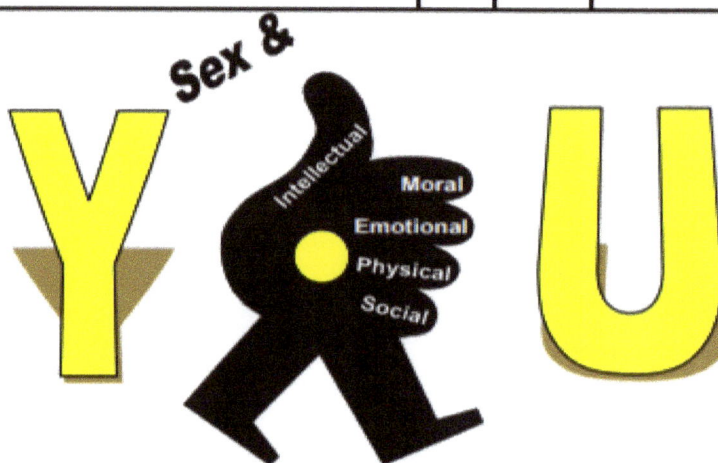

Rate the Presenters

Rate the Presenters - Put an X under your choice for each comment.	Fair	Good	Excellent
1. Presenters were knowledgeable about the Sexual Health information shared.			
2. Presenters shared the information in an understandable manner.			
3. Presenters had a caring attitude toward the students.			

Concepts of Sexual Health

Appendix Lesson 6

SH Evaluation Totals Page

Name of Presenter (s) _____ Date_____

Phone _____ Email _____

Name of School _____ Class Period _____
Teachers _____

Total Students in Class   Class Start Date _____
                                  End Date _____

         Boys   _____

         Girls   _____

Total Students   _____

% of Students Committed To Purity (No. 1 under Rate SH Program)

% Agree	Agree	Disagree	Undecided
_____ Boys			
_____ Girls			
Totals			
Total % of students Committed to Purity	%		

% of Students that would Recommend SH (No. 2 under Rate SH Program)

% Agree	Agree	Disagree	Undecided
_____ Boys			
_____ Girls			
Totals			
Total % of students Recommended SH	%		

_____
Signature of Presenter

Available for future presentations?   Y   N   If yes, days available   M   T   W   T   F
                                                                       (Circle)

Notes

[1] Arkansas State Health Profile http://www.cdc.gov/nchhstp/stateprofiles/pdf/arkansas_profile.pdf

[2] Onalee McGraw, Teaching the Whole Person about Love, Sex and Marriage, Educating for Character in the Common World of our Homes, Schools and Communities (Educational Guidance Institute, Front Royal, Virginia, 2004), 43.

[3] Concepts of Sexual Health, Sex & You Curriculum, (Concepts of Truth, Inc., 2010, 2015, 2018 Revised)

[4] Love & Life at the Movies: Growing in Love with the Film Classics, (Educational Guidance Institute, Front Royal, Virginia, 2008)

[5] Pam Stenzel, The High Cost of Free Love, (www.pamstenzel.com, 2012)

[6] McDowell, Josh, "Rules Without Relationships=Rebellion", Frequently Asked Questions, http://www.josh.org

[7] Onalee McGraw, Teaching the Whole Person about Love, Sex and Marriage, Educating for Character in the Common World of our Homes, Schools and Communities (Educational Guidance Institute, Front Royal, Virginia, 2004), 52.

[8] Ibid, 51.

[9] Ibid, 51.

[10] WHO World Health Organization definition of Sexual Health, 2002

[11] Onalee McGraw, Teaching the Whole Person about Love, Sex and Marriage, Educating for Character in the Common World of our Homes, Schools and Communities (Educational Guidance Institute, Front Royal, Virginia, 2004),12

[12] J. Budziszewski, "What We Lose When We Forget What Sex Is For", (Fellowship of St. James, 2005), http://www.Touchstonemag.com/archives/print.php

[13] Ibid.

[14] "Hardwired to Connect: The New Scientific Case for Authoritative Communities. (New York: Institute for American Values, 2003), 31-32

[15] Bill & Pam Farrel, Men Are Like Waffles, Women Are Like Spaghetti (Harvest House Publishers, 2007)

[16] Budziszewski, J., "What We Lose When We Forget What Sex Is For", (Fellowship of St. James, 2005), http://www. Touchstonemag.com/archives/print.php

[17] "Universal Declaration of Human Rights",1948, http://www.un.org/en/documents/udhr/

[18] Budziszewski, J., "What We Lose When We Forget What Sex Is For", (Fellowship of St. James, 2005), http://www. Touchstonemag.com/archives/print.php

[19] Ibid.

[20] Ibid.

[21] Barbara Wilson, The Invisible Bond, (Colorado Springs, Co: Multnomah Books, 2006), 30-33

[22] "Science of Sex", http://www.humanlife.org/onlinecitations.php

[23] "Secondary Virginity", Concepts of Truth, Inc. Appendix, Lesson 1, 2018

[24] "Science of Sex", http://www.humanlife.org/onlinecitations.php

[25] Joe S. McIlhaney, Jr., M.D., Freda McKissic Bush, M.D., Hooked, New Science On How Casual Sex Is Affecting Our Children, (Northfield Publishing, Chicago, Illinois, 2008)

R. E. Rector, K. A. Johnson, and L. R. Noyes, "Sexually Active Teenagers Are More Likely to Be Depressed and to Attempt Suicide," Washington D.C.: A report from the Heritage Center for Data Analysis, "The Heritage Foundation. Publication CDA03-04, June 2 (2005)

Barnet et al., 2004; Breheny & Stephens, 2007; Forum on Child & Family Statistics, 2007; Hofferth et al., 2001; Hoffman, 2006, Pregnancy and Childbearing Among U.S. Teens http://www.planned-parenthoodnj.org/library/topic/family_planning/teen_pregnancy

 L. Coley and P. L. Chase-Lansdale, "Adolescent Pregnancy and Parenthood: Recent Evidence and Future Directions," American Psychologist 53, no. 2 (1998): 152-166.

Nicole M. Else-Quest, Janet Shibley Hyde, and John D. DeLamater, "Context Counts: Long-Term Sequelae of Pre-marital Intercourse or Abstinence", The Journal of Sex Research, Vol. 42, 2005

Lee A. Lillard, Michael J. Brien, and Linda J. Eaite, "Pre-Marital Cohabitation and Subsequent Marital Dissolution: Is It Self-Selection?" Demography 32 (1995): 437-458.

Elizabeth Thomsom and Ugo Collela, "Cohabitation and Marital Stability: Quality or Commitment?" Journal of Marriage and the Family 54 (1992): 259-268.

G. K. Rhoades, S. M. Stanley, H. J. Markman, "Pre-engagement cohabitation and gender asymmetry in marital commitment," Journal of Family Psychology (Dec. 2006): 20 (4):553-60.

C. T. Kenney, S. S. McLanahan, "Why are cohabitating relationships more violent than marriages?" Demography (Feb. 2006): 43 (1): 127-40

Harvard University Study "Dad is Destiny", U.S. News and World Report, (Feb. 27, 1995)

[26] Bill & Pam Farel, Men Are Like Waffles, Women Are Like Spaghetti (Harvest House Publishers, 2007)

[27] TED: Alexander Tsiaras, (The Ink Conference, 2010)

[28] J. Budziszewski, "What We Lose When We Forget What Sex Is For", (Fellowship of St. James, 2005),   http://www. Touchstonemag.com/archives/print.php

[29] Horton Hears a Who!, (2008), http://en.wikiquote.org/wiki/Horton_Hears_a_Who!_(film)

[30] TED: Alexander Tsiaras, (The Ink Conference, 2010)

[31] Touch of Life Fetal Models, (Heritage House'76, Inc., Snowflake, Arizona)

[32] Scott Klusendorf, S.L.E.D.,(Stand to Reason), http://www.str.org

[33] "Universal Declaration of Human Rights", 1948, http://www.un.org/en/documents/udhr/

[34] Universal Declaration of Human Rights Animated Version, http://www.youtube.com, Oct 15, 2008

[35] " Love & Life at the Movies: Growing in Love with the Film Classics Roman Holiday Love and Responsibility", (Educational Guidance Institute, 2008)

[36] Ibid.

[37] If it's not OK for him to take steroids...why is it OK for her? by Breast Cancer Prevention Institute   http://www.bcpinstitute.org

[38] Drs. John and Evelyn Billings, The Billings Ovulation Method™, http://www.billingslife.org

[39] Sexual Exposure Chart, wvdhhr.org/.../edresources/sexual_exposure_chart.pdf

[40] STD Test, (Concepts of Truth International, 2015, 2018 Revised)

[41] Ibid.

[42] Ibid.

[43] Pam Stenzel, Leader's Guide and Student Handouts for Sex, Love Relationships, Straight Talk on Teen Sexuality, (Gateway Films Vision Video, Worchester, PA), 36

[44] Pam Stenzel, The High Cost of Free Love, (www.pamstenzel.com, 2012)

[45] Ibid.

[46] Ibid.

www.ingramcontent.com/pod-product-compliance
Lightning Source LLC
Chambersburg PA
CBHW051557030426

42334CB00034B/3468